Contents

Introduction

The aim of this book is to provide the reader with the knowledge required to assess children for possible signs and symptoms of illness so that they can be given the care and treatment needed. Although the book has been written to meet the requirements of the NVQ, CACHE and BTEC diploma syllabuses, its content will also be recommended reading for anyone involved in the care of children including parents, older siblings and baby sitters.

Children often find it difficult to interpret the feelings they have and their language ability will limit communication of how they feel. They may be unable to make any sense of these feelings as they have little understanding of how their body works. It is for these reasons that they may not always give the warning signs so readily vocalised by adults whenever they feel unwell, and it is therefore up to the carers to be alert enough to notice the subtle changes that might indicate illness.

The book takes the reader from discussions on health and its meaning through to ill health, its identification and the possible clues children might give when unwell. Caring for children and its effect on the carer, are explored, along with the various categories of ill health. The introduction of each gives the reader an outline of the information included with cross-referencing to other chapters being made clear when appropriate.

Throughout the book the carers and children are referred to as 'she'. The intention is not to suggest that carers are only female – indeed I would support moves to involve more men in child care – or that sick children are only female. It simply served to avoid the somewhat cumbersome 'he or she' or even 's/he' and will, I hope, make the reading smoother.

The following terms have been used throughout the book: *carer* – describes the person caring for the child, either early years worker or parent; *early years worker* – describes a carer who is not a parent to the child; *parent* – when only a parent would be in the situation.

Activities are included in all chapters: their aim is to broaden the possible areas of enquiry.

1

Exploration of Health

The early years worker will usually care for well and healthy children; however, it is important that she is able to recognise some of the signs and symptoms that suggest children are ill. Thus, she can contact a child's parents who may take over the caring role.

Her role in the recognition of a very ill child may be vitally important. It may be that the child becomes rapidly unwell, as in conditions such as meningitis, where medical help is urgently required.

In order to be able to recognise ill health, the early years worker needs to have a clear notion of what is meant by 'health' and 'ill health' so that she can ensure that children have the very best of care at all times.

This chapter seeks to discuss the notions of health and ill health.

What is health?

ACTIVITY

Defining health is not as straightforward as it might first appear and it is worth reflecting on your own understanding. Write down how you would describe health and ask colleagues or your relatives how they would describe it. Use these notes to compare with the following text.

Undoubtedly health means different things to different people, therefore identifying a comprehensive definition is somewhat difficult. No one definition seems to be wholly acceptable.

The general public may not give much consideration to their health until they become ill (despite the fact that increasingly we are being encouraged to take responsibility for our own health). If this is the case then they might be hard pressed to define health but find ill health a much easier concept to explain.

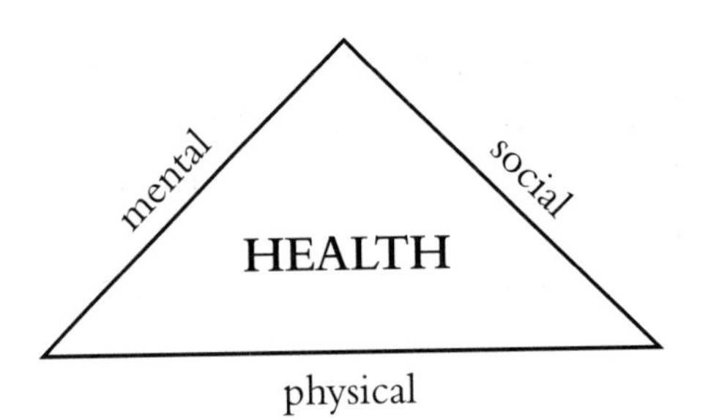

Figure 1 The three aspects of health

In 1948 the World Health Organisation (WHO) defined health as being 'a state of complete physical, mental and social well-being and not merely the absence of disease or infirmity'.

This definition is somewhat idealistic and the reader could be excused for wondering if there is anyone who could actually be described as being healthy. However, what this definition does provide is a framework for health. It has three facets, physical, mental and social, and these may be diagrammatically represented as shown in Figure 1.

- *Physical health* is concerned with the physical and mechanical functioning of the body, such as walking.
- *Mental health* is the ability to think clearly, to make judgements and to cope with the effects of daily life.
- *Social health* is concerned with the ability to relate to other people and to make and maintain relationships.

The WHO definition does not take into account the environmental, emotional and spiritual factors that are also considered to be part of the framework of health. Figure 2 shows how representation may now be seen when these are noted.

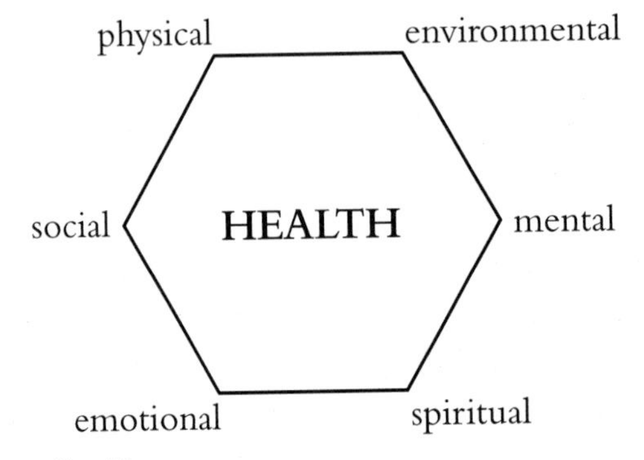

Figure 2 The six aspects of health

- *Emotional health* is concerned with the ability to express emotion and to cope with adverse conditions, such as stress.
- *Spiritual health* may be concerned with religious practices and beliefs and/or moral issues.
- *Environmental health* is concerned not only with the physical environment but also the health of the society in which the person lives.

If individuals are to achieve and maintain a healthy state then they will need to be active in its pursuit; for instance, taking regular exercise, developing friendships and strategies for coping with adverse stressful situations.

Examples of factors that influence health can be listed as follows:

Physical	Mental	Social	Environmental	Spiritual	Emotional
exercise, balanced diet	stimulation, relaxation	friendship	clean air, clean water	inner peace, sense of fulfilment	strategies for coping with stress

However, it should be noted that factors that affect health cannot always be neatly categorised. For example, suitable housing may appear under physical, mental, social and environmental headings as it has an effect on more than one aspect of health.

ACTIVITY

Together with a group of colleagues expand the examples shown above to produce a fuller list of influences on health.

The carer as a role model

Children need to be involved in the pursuit of health from an early age. They are, however, very dependent on their carers for guidance and support if they are to achieve the goal.

Adults have a responsibility to ensure a positive influence on the health and well-being of children in their care. It will be recalled that learning takes place in various ways; some through observation of adult patterns of behaviour (modelling). It is therefore important that adults provide a consistently high standard from which children can learn.

ACTIVITY

List the ways in which you think children could possibly learn and imitate healthy pursuits from you.

Now list the ways in which children could learn unhealthy pursuits from you. Take this second list and work out a strategy of either giving up these pursuits or of ensuring children do not observe you doing them. For example, if you are a smoker ideally you might like to think about giving up, or, if not, you should not smoke anywhere near children.

What is ill health?

Ill health refers to the subjective feeling of loss of health. From experience adults can interpret the characteristics suggestive of ill health, for instance a headache, aching limbs and a raised temperature may suggest a bout of the 'flu. Children with less experience and linguistic ability might behave differently and become clingy or whiny. The carer will need to 'tune in' to changes in behaviour, particularly when they are associated with other non-verbal cues that suggest children are unwell. As children get older and gain experience they will learn to associate these feelings with loss of health and to express these feelings verbally.

Ill health is often used interchangeably with the term 'disease'. However, disease refers to an objective state of ill health whereby there is some malfunctioning of the body, for example children who have the disease chickenpox will show specific signs and symptoms and will feel ill.

Some diseases are preventable, for example cholera (an infectious disease responsible for many deaths in the nineteenth century) can be prevented by the provision of a clean water supply. Many other infectious diseases can be prevented by immunisation.

Disease, particularly long-term, may affect the growth and development of children and this is often identified at the child surveillance clinic.

ACTIVITY

Reference has been made to non-verbal cues that might suggest ill health. Using a spider diagram format, develop a diagram with your colleagues to include all the non-verbal cues that might be shown.

Ill health often affects more than one area of health. For instance, the alcoholic may have high blood pressure and be susceptible to infections (physical), have delusions (mental), be isolated (social) and these factors may result in stress, further compounding the problem.

Conclusion

The early years worker, through working closely with the children in her care, can 'tune in' to individuals and can therefore often detect small changes in behaviour which may suggest ill health. This is a valuable skill which can be developed through the numerous child observations she undertakes during training. Child observations should form an integral part of ongoing professional development.

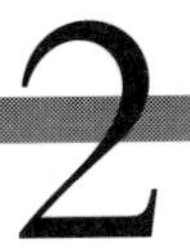

Influences on Health

> The promotion of child health requires a shift in the relationship between parents, children and health professionals to one of partnership rather than supervision, in which parents are empowered to make use of services and expertise according to their needs (Hall, 1996).

Health is influenced by many factors and does not occur as the result of luck. The early years worker, who has a knowledge of factors that may influence health, will be able to work towards ensuring her own good health and that of the children in her care. It is essential that she continues to read widely on health issues both during training and as part of professional development thereafter.

Hall (as quoted above) highlights the important issues of partnership, and the early years worker should be included within this partnership. She will need to liaise with the parents on a regular basis and health professionals on an occasional basis.

The four main influences on health

ACTIVITY

Before reading further, consider factors that you think influence your personal health. Consider these in terms of personal factors, factors in your immediate environment such as home or college, and factors that are found in the wider environment such as air quality. Write these down and compare them with the following text.

Factors that influence health may be grouped into four main areas:

- biological
- environmental
- lifestyle
- social.

Biological

These factors relate to the processes within the body, that is, the biological make up of the individual, and includes inherited factors (genetic factors). Man is a complex organism and this complexity can contribute to illness and disease. Children will inherit factors from both parents and these will influence their health either beneficially or adversely.

Biological factors include susceptibility to disease. Several diseases can now be prevented by the widespread availability, in many countries, of immunisations which are effective against infectious diseases such as measles, mumps and rubella.

Recent medical advances in gene therapy have the potential to reduce or possibly eradicate certain hereditary conditions in the future. The role of the genetic counsellor has empowered couples to make informed decisions when there is a defective gene within the family.

Environmental

These factors are external to the body and individuals may have little control over them. They include:

- *Water supply*
  Many micro-organisms are found in unclean water and once ingested can lead to human infections. Occasional spells of dry weather in the UK have led to periodic health warnings telling people to boil tap water before drinking it. Fortunately these occurrences are uncommon in the UK but in many parts of the world water supplies are sources of infection.
- *Sewage and waste removal*
  It is vital that good sanitation is achieved to help prevent the spread of disease. Micro-organisms thrive in waste matter, which often provides ideal conditions for their growth and multiplication.
- *Air*
  Several contaminants in the air including chemicals, ozone and dust, may contribute to ill health. The link between breathing in the smoke of someone else's cigarette (passive smoking) and health has become apparent over recent years and children are particularly vulnerable, presenting with conditions such as asthma.

Lifestyle

This section on lifestyle factors is not exhaustive, but serves to provide some examples. These factors include the health behaviour of individuals, and children will be influenced to a large extent by the health behaviour of their carers. Lifestyle factors include:

- *Smoking*
  Smoking is a behaviour that adversely affects the health of both active smokers and passive non-smokers who have to inhale the smoke from others' cigarettes.
  Long-term effects of smoking include coronary heart disease, increased risks of developing cancers, particularly of the lungs but also of the stomach, oesophagus, bladder and cervix.
  If a woman smokes during pregnancy her baby has a greater risk of cot death. There is also an increased risk of the baby being born prematurely and of low birth weight, as well as an increased risk of foetal and neonatal death after exposure to cigarette smoke in pregnancy.
  Research has shown that children exposed to cigarette smoke during childhood are more likely to develop glue ear, asthma, and have an increased risk of being admitted to hospital as a result of respiratory infections.
  Research has also shown there is an increased risk of children taking up the smoking habit if one or both of the parents smoke, and this is an important issue for parents and early years workers to consider. It is therefore extremely important that adults are aware of the possible harm done by smoking and to avoid taking children into smoky environments as much as is possible.
- *Diet*
  Food is needed by the body for growth and repair and energy. It is important that children develop healthy eating habits as research has shown that such habits developed in childhood are likely to be retained into adult life.
  The carer must have a good working knowledge of dietary requirements and the constituents of a balanced diet. See the section on 'Diet' in Chapter 3.
- *Exercise*
  The greatest single health risk in Britain today is coronary heart disease. Research has shown that physically inactive people have approximately double the chance of suffering from coronary heart disease.
  Research has also shown that there are more inactive girls than boys in Britain, but that there are still substantial numbers of both. There is

evidence that children who exercise become adults who exercise. It is therefore important that the carer encourages children to be active.

Exercise is beneficial both to children and adults. It has a 'feel-good' effect, allowing the individual to feel more relaxed and able to cope with life's stresses. This is just as important for children as for adults. Children can 'run off' their pent-up feelings of aggression through play and exercise.

Exercise allows children to develop fine and gross motor skills, it allows them to feel more confident with their bodies and helps social skills when undertaken in groups.

Social

The social class to which an individual is said to belong is based on the Registrar General's scale of occupational classes. These occupational classes are divided as follows:

Social class		Examples of occupations
I	Professional	doctor, lawyer
II	Intermediate	teacher, nurse, manager
IIIN	Skilled non-manual	shop assistant, clerical worker, secretary
IIIM	Skilled manual	bus driver, butcher
IV	Semi-skilled	bus conductor, postman
V	Unskilled	labourer, cleaner

The social class into which the child is born reflects the living standards, way of life and the health status of the family.

Inequalities in health were highlighted in 1980 when the Black Report was published. This report showed that those in social class I were found to have the best health status and those in social class V had the worst health status. There was a gradual decline from social class I to social class V. Furthermore, for almost every illness and disability those in the higher social classes faired better than those in the lower social classes.

Despite the Black Report highlighting the problem, eight years later the Health Divide was published and this report confirmed the original findings and showed that in some places the inequalities had become greater.

Arising from the research there are three main social factors linked to health:

- *Employment*
  Some occupations carry a higher risk to health, for instance there may

be an increased risk of accidents, stress or exposure to noise in some factories which in turn may lead to health problems.

Unemployment has been shown to adversely affect health, with those who are unemployed having a higher incidence of mental ill health, long-term physical illness, disability and higher mortality rates.

ACTIVITY

'Unemployment has been shown to adversely affect health.' In what ways does unemployment affect the health of children? You are advised to think in terms of the various aspects of health, physical, social, mental, etc. and to use these as a basis for developing this piece of work which should be presented in a spider diagram format.

- *Income*
  The level of income will determine the resources available to the family and will affect housing, diet, and have an impact on social support. In general, the lower the social class, the lower the income and the poorer the health.
  Provision of housing and food will absorb a large proportion of the family income and may leave little over. Studies have shown that the diet of poorer people is less healthy than those who are better off.
  Poverty is associated with ill health and it is difficult to escape from the poverty trap.
- *Housing*
  Housing has an effect on health and this may be seen most profoundly in the health of homeless people who are at risk from accidents, depression and infectious diseases.
  In general, those in lower social classes live in poorer housing and in more crowded conditions than those who are better off. Poor housing and overcrowding can have a profound effect on the physical, mental, social and emotional well-being of the family.

ACTIVITY

'Poor housing and overcrowding can have a profound effect on the physical, mental, social and emotional well-being of the family.' Discuss this statement with your colleagues, and make a note of your discussions using a spider diagram format, one for each aspect of health.

Cultural effects

Britain is a multicultural society and cultural differences between groups may have a bearing on their attitudes towards health. Early years workers need to be sensitive to the beliefs and attitudes held by children and their families. They should strive to work together, exchanging information to avoid conflict.

Conclusion

This chapter began with a quote highlighting the importance of developing a partnership between the parents, children and health professionals for the sake of children's health. Early years workers can also develop this partnership and foster positive influences which may lead to children developing into healthier adults.

3

Maintenance of Personal Health

Caring for children is extremely demanding work and its value should never be underestimated. Carers have a responsibility to look after their children to the very best of their ability and to recognise the importance of maintaining their own health so that they can fulfil this role. If individuals are to achieve and maintain a healthy state then they will need to be active in its pursuit.

Factors that promote health

- **Physical** factors include taking exercise, eating a balanced diet and getting sufficient sleep.
- **Mental** factors include allowing sufficient time for relaxation and controlling stress.
- Within **social** factors consideration must be given to developing social contacts, developing social and interpersonal skills, not smoking, alcohol intake, practising safe sex (if appropriate).
- **Environmental** factors include good housing and sanitation, high standards of hygiene and providing a safe environment.
- **Spiritual** factors include finding inner peace and contentment which may or may not include practising religion.
- **Emotional** factors include recognition and management of stress.

Each of these factors will be considered in more detail.

Exercise

Taking regular exercise has benefits, in terms of health and well-being, to children and adults. It has a 'feel-good' effect, allowing the individual to feel more relaxed and able to cope with the strains of life, which is just as important for children as for adults. Children can 'run off' their pent-up feelings of aggression through play and exercise.

There are four main benefits of taking exercise:

- **Suppleness.** If joints and muscles are not exercised they become stiff and ultimately movement becomes restricted. Regular exercise results

in the ability to take exercise without stiffness and prevents problems later in life.
- **Strength.** Inactive muscles waste if they are not regularly exercised. This can be readily demonstrated by observation of a limb just after the removal of a plaster of Paris when the underlying muscles have not been adequately exercised. Regular exercise maintains the size and efficiency of muscles.
- **Stamina.** Taking regular exercise increases the efficiency of the heart and lungs and therefore allows the individual to exercise without feeling uncomfortably breathless.
- **Skill and co-ordination.** Taking regular exercise allows the body to be used confidently.

Coronary heart disease is the greatest single health risk to adults in Britain today. According to research physically inactive people have approximately double the chance of suffering from this. The heart itself is a muscle and needs to be exercised regularly. Current recommendations from the Health Education Authority (HEA) are that adults should take thirty minutes of exercise five times a week; it does not have to be rigorous exercise, simply enough to cause the breathing rate to increase slightly.

ACTIVITY

Read the leaflets on exercise produced by the HEA, some of which may be found in health centres or you could write to the HEA (address on page 217). Discuss with colleagues how you might be able to incorporate its recommendations into your daily life.

Children need to take regular physical activity and time should be incorporated into the day to allow for this. In addition to the benefits discussed, it allows opportunities for **social interaction**, for example, children can meet other children at the park or swimming pool. This also provides an opportunity for carers to meet others. It should be remembered that all too often the benefits of walking are overlooked and the car is used for unnecessary journeys.

ACTIVITY

Research the possibilities in your area for taking exercise: list the parks and playgrounds within walking distance, find out the whereabouts of the local swimming pool and any leisure centre activities for children both in term time and in the school holidays.

Diet

Food provides energy and is required for growth and repair of tissues. A balanced diet is essential for good health and is achieved by eating the correct types of food, in sufficient quantities, according to age, sex, body size and occupation. Too much will ultimately lead to obesity and too little to loss of weight. Both of these states are unhealthy.

Components of a balanced diet include:

- proteins
- carbohydrates
- fats
- minerals
- vitamins
- fibre
- water.

These components can be grouped in the following way:

- Group 1 Bread, pasta, potatoes, cereals, rice.
- Group 2 Fruit and vegetables (current recommendations from the HEA are that we should eat five portions a day).
- Group 3 Milk and milk products.
- Group 4 High protein foods.
- Group 5 Fats and oils.

A balanced diet means eating some foods from each of these groups, however it is important that proportions are taken into account. Foods from group 1 should form the major input of the diet and those in group 5 should be taken in small amounts. This can be represented as shown in Figure 3.

ACTIVITY

Using library facilities list several examples of each food group.

Over the next week keep a diary of all the food and drink you consume. On a daily basis try to break down each meal into its components.

Sitting down to eat as a family helps to shape children's eating habits, for example, if they observe people they know eating healthy foods such as salads, or not adding salt or sugar to foods, they will follow the example.

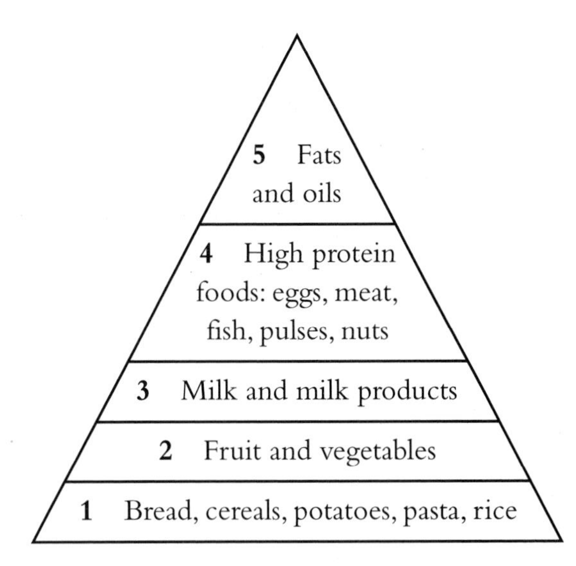

Figure 3 Recommendations for a healthy diet

Carers should have a good understanding of dietary requirements so that they can ensure the child is given a balanced diet.

ACTIVITY

Using library facilities, list the possible food sources of vitamins A, B, C, D, E and K, and the minerals calcium, iron, copper and zinc.

List the possible deficiency disorders for the above vitamins and minerals.

Sleep and relaxation

Adequate sleep is essential for health. The amount needed varies with each individual and there are no hard and fast rules on the amount that should be taken. It is important that as far as possible the individual acknowledges their own requirements and takes as much sleep as is needed. Young children require more sleep than adults, and carers should 'tune' into their needs.

Both adults and children must have some time for relaxation to unwind from the stresses and strains of the day. This may take whatever form suits the individual, such as reading, listening to music or watching television.

Stress

Stress may be caused by any event that results in anger, irritation, tension or frustration. Factors that cause stress in one person may excite another and therefore individuals need to learn to recognise their own stressors and avoid them or learn coping strategies. It is recognised that high levels of stress without any method of coping can lead to physical and mental ill health.

Coping strategies may include taking regular exercise or ensuring enough relaxation time is built into the day. Carers not only need to recognise their own stress and stressors but also those that cause stress in the children they care for. Children are also prone to stress resulting from insufficient time for relaxation or picking up on the stresses of the family environment.

ACTIVITY

List factors in your life that cause anger, irritation, tension or frustration. Identify which factors cause the most stress and try to identify ways of lessening the effect. It may be helpful to discuss this activity with your friends or colleagues.

Social contacts

People are generally sociable creatures and need to make and develop friendships and working relationships with others. Adults usually value friendships from which they may derive support and encouragement.

Children will play alongside other children from the age of two years and will later play with other children. Interaction with children and adults allows them to develop a sense of identity and self-esteem. In the early years and school settings children learn the importance of behaving as expected, sharing and generally getting along with other adults and children.

Smoking

Smoking is the United Kingdom's largest single preventable cause of premature death. It is a behaviour that adversely affects the health of both smokers and non-smokers who have to endure the effects of passive smoking. Cigarette smoke contains over 4000 chemicals of which 55 are carcinogenic (cause cancer). These chemicals are found within the three main components of cigarettes: nicotine, carbon monoxide and tar.

There is a strong link between children who passively smoke and ill health. Research shows a link between exposure to cigarette smoke during pregnancy and increased risks of foetal and neonatal death, prematurity and low birth weight. Passive smoking has been linked to asthma and cot death. It is estimated that a large number of adult deaths from coronary heart disease are linked to cigarette smoking. Smoking is also linked to cancer of the lungs and other cancers, bronchitis, strokes, etc.

Research has shown that children of parents who smoke are more likely to want to smoke themselves. Therefore, it follows that if the carer does smoke, they should stop or at least not smoke in the presence of children.

Alcohol

Many adults enjoy a drink and drinking within the 'sensible limit', as recommended by the government, can have some health benefits. However, drinking in quantities beyond these limits may adversely affect health.

In order to stay within the sensible limits carers must understand the measurement of alcohol (units) in order to keep a tally of the amount consumed.

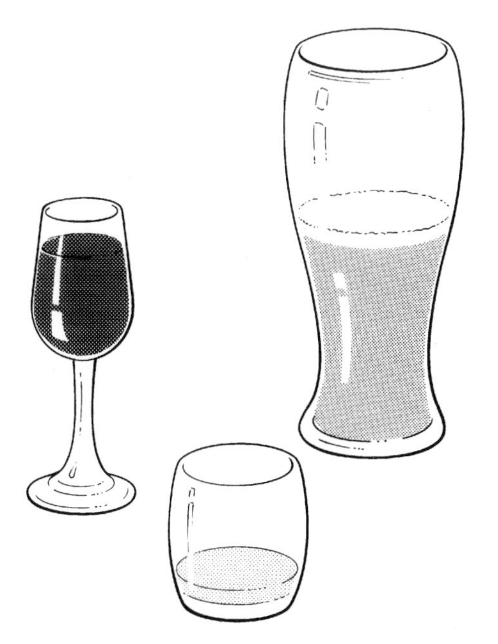

Figure 4 Each drink shown is equal to one unit of alcohol: one glass of wine, a single measure of spirits, half a pint of beer

ACTIVITY

Using library facilities find out the current recommendations for 'sensible drinking'.

Carers should refrain from drinking during the day as alcohol may affect concentration and put children at risk. Alcohol must be kept out of the reach of children as even small amounts can have adverse effects.

Sexual practices

Sexually active adults should practise safe sex which includes using a condom when having intercourse, keeping the number of sexual partners to a minimum and knowing their sexual history. Safe sex allows individuals to avoid sexually transmitted diseases including HIV/AIDS, and unwanted pregnancy.

Housing and the provision of a safe environment

The individual's basic needs include food, shelter and warmth, all of which should be provided by housing of a good standard and appropriate for the climate. Consideration needs to be given to the insulation of the house, maintenance of an adequate temperature both in the winter and the summer, effective ventilation, adequate lighting, a good clean water supply, effective sanitation (removal of sewage and refuse collection), the surrounding environment (including accessibility to shops, a transport system and play areas) and the provision within the home of a supporting atmosphere in which the individual members can relax and feel safe. It is also necessary to consider the size of the accommodation and to avoid overcrowding as this can lead to health problems, such as spread of infection. (The final Activity in Chapter 2 highlights how housing may be associated with poor health.)

Inherent within the housing issue is the importance of practising a high standard of hygiene and providing a safe environment. These issues will now be considered.

PERSONAL CLEANLINESS

The carer needs to remember that children learn, in part, through modelling themselves on adults and it is therefore essential that the role model practises a high standard of hygiene for the child to copy. See Figure 5.

KITCHEN CLEANLINESS

A multitude of germs and other dangers to children can be found in the kitchen. Figure 6 on page 20 highlights some which the carer should pay particular attention to.

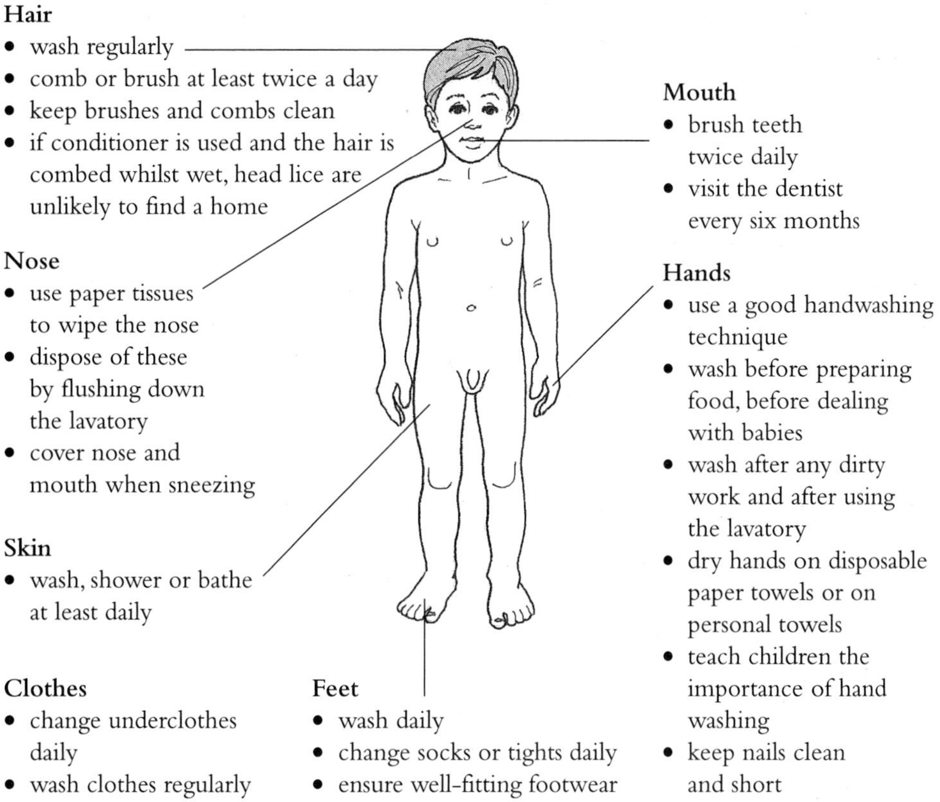

Hair
- wash regularly
- comb or brush at least twice a day
- keep brushes and combs clean
- if conditioner is used and the hair is combed whilst wet, head lice are unlikely to find a home

Nose
- use paper tissues to wipe the nose
- dispose of these by flushing down the lavatory
- cover nose and mouth when sneezing

Skin
- wash, shower or bathe at least daily

Clothes
- change underclothes daily
- wash clothes regularly

Feet
- wash daily
- change socks or tights daily
- ensure well-fitting footwear

Mouth
- brush teeth twice daily
- visit the dentist every six months

Hands
- use a good handwashing technique
- wash before preparing food, before dealing with babies
- wash after any dirty work and after using the lavatory
- dry hands on disposable paper towels or on personal towels
- teach children the importance of hand washing
- keep nails clean and short

Figure 5 Recommendations for personal cleanliness

CLEANLINESS IN THE HOME/WORKPLACE

Within the main caring environment the following areas should be attended to:

- Carpets should be vacuumed frequently.
- Floors should be washed frequently.
- Toilets, baths and basins should be cleaned frequently.
- Toys and playthings should be washed frequently.

ANIMALS

Animals can expose children to a number of health threats:

- Animal excreta in the garden should be disposed of in a place that is inaccessible to children.
- Care should be taken when dealing with cat litter trays. They should be changed daily and must be left where they are inaccessible to children.
- Cats and dogs should be regularly wormed.
- Unwell animals should be seen by a vet.

Ventilation
- open the window to ventilate the kitchen

Sink
- wash hands before and after food preparation
- wash cutlery and crockery thoroughly using hot water

General hygiene
- keep animals out of the kitchen

Sterilising unit
- bottles and dummies must be sterilised. Immerse them for the required time
- change sterilising fluid daily

Surfaces
- clean surfaces daily, always before and after food preparation, and after placing shopping bags on the surfaces

Waste bin
- empty regularly and wash as necessary

Floor
- wash the floor regularly
- mop up spillages straight away

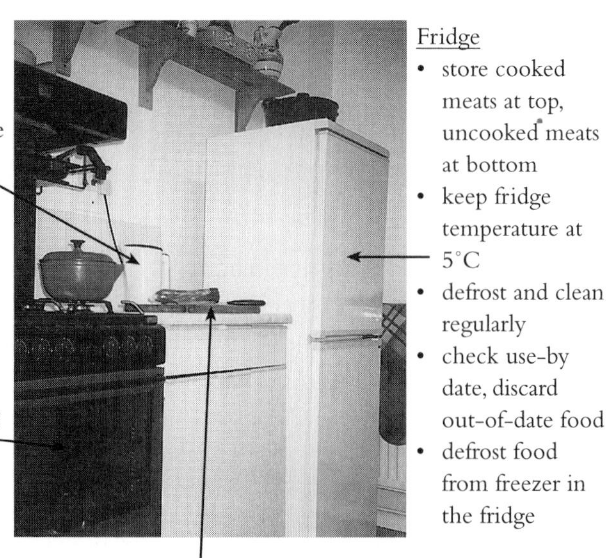

Electrical appliances
- keep flexes away from edge of surfaces

Cooking
- cook food thoroughly
- avoid reheating food

Fridge
- store cooked meats at top, uncooked meats at bottom
- keep fridge temperature at 5°C
- defrost and clean regularly
- check use-by date, discard out-of-date food
- defrost food from freezer in the fridge

Chopping boards
- keep separate boards for meat and vegetable preparation

Figure 6 Kitchen cleanliness

Providing a safe environment

The carer has a responsibility to prevent accidents as far as possible, and to ensure this it is essential that she attempts to see the world through the eyes of the child. (Providing a safe environment is further discussed in Chapter 16.)

Spiritual factors

Inner peace and contentment, which may or may not include practising religion, is a personal aspect of health for which there are no hard and fast guidelines.

Conclusion

If individuals are to attain their potential health status there is no room for complacency. Beneficial and perhaps some adverse factors may have been inherited from parents but it is up to individuals to make the very best of these and strive for personal health. Empowerment is the key – if individuals have the knowledge and understanding they can make the most of the resources available to them to achieve the goal of health.

4

Measurement of Health

In 1901 the life expectancy in the United Kingdom at birth was 45.5 years for a boy and 49 years for a girl. In 1991 the life expectancy at birth was 73.2 years for a boy and 78.8 years for a girl. During this period there has been a dramatic decline in the number of deaths during the first year of life (infant mortality) from 142 to 7 per 1000 live births. Thus there has been a remarkable improvement in the health of those resident in the UK.

ACTIVITY

List any factors that you think may have contributed to the improvements in health.

Both infant mortality and life expectancy figures are a good indicator of the health profile of a nation. The improvements in the health profile of the UK have arisen for a number of reasons. Infections were a major cause of death (mortality) and ill health (morbidity) in the UK. The nineteenth century saw high levels of mortality and morbidity from infectious diseases such as tuberculosis, cholera, typhoid and measles, whilst since 1900 there has been a marked decline in these diseases. This decline is attributed to immunisation programmes and to improvements in medicine with the most significant contribution being from improvements in living standards. However, alongside the decline in infectious diseases there has been an increase in the incidence of other chronic diseases such as coronary heart disease, strokes and cancers.

Provision of free health care has allowed those who previously could not afford health care to benefit. The National Health Service (NHS) provides primary health care through the health centres and secondary health care through hospitals.

Epidemiology

An epidemic is the widespread occurrence of a disease at a particular time.

Epidemiology is the study of factors affecting disease in a given population. It is important to study such factors, because information gathered on aspects of child health assist in planning health care provision, preventing illness and controlling the spread of illness.

Epidemiologists study groups of individuals (populations) to investigate the numbers affected by an aspect of health. Information needs to be collected from a cross-section of people, both healthy and sick, in order to determine the numbers of ill people in a given population. This information may be collected nationally or locally, depending on the nature of the study. It can, for instance, be collected routinely from registration of births and deaths, or the information can be collected by the population census every ten years or by specific surveys set up to study a specific population or disease, as in the Black Report (1980) referred to in Chapter 2. Information is published yearly via the Office of Population Censuses and Surveys (OPCS), and includes information on the social class of those surveyed, their age and causes of death. It is divided into sections on mortality and morbidity.

Mortality

This is information gathered on numbers and causes of death. Infant and perinatal mortality rates are indicators of the health status of a population.

INFANT MORTALITY RATE

This is the number of deaths of infants under the age of one year per 1000 live births.

Note: the infant mortality rate of children born into families of social class V (unskilled workers) is twice that of children born to social class I (professional families).

PERINATAL MORTALITY RATE

This is the number of stillbirths (death of the foetus after the twenty-eighth week of pregnancy) and deaths that occur within the first week of life.

Note: the perinatal mortality rate of children born to social class V (unskilled workers) is more than three times greater than children born to social class I (professional families).

NEONATAL MORTALITY RATE

The number of deaths within the first four weeks of life. The common causes of death during this period are related to immaturity, congenital abnormalities and infections.

MATERNAL MORTALITY RATE

The number of deaths of women associated with childbirth per 1000 births. Maternal mortality rates have fallen since 1935.

Morbidity

This is information on illness, whether caused by disease, injury or disability. However, it is more difficult to collect information on morbidity, because the collection relies on reports from many sources, and not all cases are reported. Morbidity is measured as prevalence (the proportion of a group of people having a condition at any one time) and incidence (the number of new cases reported within a stated time).

Information can be collected via the census and through notification of certain infectious diseases which have to be reported. General practitioners, hospitals and social security departments keep various registers which provide information for the surveys, such as the child protection register.

With increasing computerisation, information gathering should become easier and more reliable.

Conclusion

The twentieth century has seen a significant improvement in health, as the result of several factors. It is important that information on health and ill health is collected and analysed to assist in the pursuit of further improvements and adequate health care provisions for the future.

5

Child Health Promotion

Carers are invited to bring children to the child health clinic (sometimes called the child surveillance clinic) at regular intervals during their early years. These clinics aim to:

- promote health and prevent illness
- allow early detection of problems and abnormalities and therefore offer early treatment.

Promotion of health and prevention of illness

Health promotion is when individuals are empowered through planned and informed intervention to improve their health or to prevent illness. Health professionals can use the clinic as an opportunity to promote health through discussions and observations of relevant issues concerning the age and stage of development of the baby or child and the relationship of the carer with the child. Further opportunities arise through conversations with other carers where sharing of information can give reassurance to those who have less experience.

Early detection of abnormalities

Early detection of abnormalities and early treatment, if appropriate, may improve the long-term prospects for health. Parents may come to terms with an abnormality more easily if it is detected early and discussion and support is offered. Early detection may enable doctors to give advice on further pregnancies.

Child health clinics achieve these aims by inviting parents to bring babies and children at regular intervals during their early years for a medical review by a doctor or a health visitor. These clinics review babies and children at:

- six-to-eight weeks
- six-to-eight months

- two years
- four years.

They are also invited to come along to these clinics for immunisations (see Chapter 11).

The philosophy of these clinics is to welcome and encourage parents to bring their children along. Some clinics will operate a 'drop in' system whereby parents attend even if they do not have an appointment, thus encouraging a supportive environment where health professionals are available for advice, alongside other parents who support each other.

Over recent years there has been a change in emphasis in health care and in particular in child health clinics. Partnership between the health professionals and the carer is increasingly encouraged.

Various health professionals may be present at the clinic, including the general practitioner, the health visitor and the school nurse. Parents may formally or informally discuss issues and thus become empowered to make informed decisions about their child's health and health care and to take more responsibility for health. These discussions with parents have a great value as it is often the parent who is the first to recognise that something is not quite right.

Early years workers also play a large part in the recognition of abnormalities. Children may be in their care for large portions of the day and since they have a great deal of experience they may be the first to suspect problems.

Personal Child Health Records

The Personal Child Health Record book is issued to parents in most, but not all, areas in Britain. It is given to parents soon after birth and it allows the parents, doctors and health visitors to maintain a record of the child's health, development and progress.

Parents are encouraged to take the record everywhere with them. If the child is taken ill when the family is away from home it will give much of the important information about the child, some of which might otherwise be forgotten in the anxiety of the moment.

ACTIVITY

Ask your health visitor if you could look at a Personal Child Health Record book. List the contents of the book. This might become a useful reference for later work.

Make a list of the safety information that is printed throughout the book. Familiarise yourself with the help and advice section.

Examination of the baby

The neonatal examination (which usually takes place within twenty-four hours of the birth) and the clinics (six-to-eight weeks, six-to-eight months, two years and 4 years) all review:

- growth (weight, height and head circumference)
- physical development
- motor development
- hearing and language
- vision
- social development.

The parents will also be encouraged to volunteer any information about the development of the baby or child, and the Personal Child Health Record book includes a page at each review for the parent to fill in.

Neonatal examination

This is carried out in a methodical but opportunistic way, for example if the baby is crying then the mouth will be examined at that point. Whilst the doctor is examining the baby she will explain what is being done and the reasons for doing it. The nature of the examination is usually relaxed enough to allow for any questions.

Each of the following are examined and the findings recorded:

- The overall appearance of the baby. This may reveal abnormalities, for instance, slanted eyes, low ears and a large bridge to the nose may indicate Down's syndrome.
- The weight of the baby is measured and recorded on a centile chart (see page 92).

- The head circumference is measured and recorded on a centile chart.
- The fontanelles (the soft spots on the baby's head where the skull is not fully formed) are examined. There are two fontanelles, the anterior and the posterior, and these should both be felt. They should feel soft to the touch and neither bulging or sunken.
- The mouth is checked for the presence of a cleft palate (a small hole in the roof of the mouth). If present, this will need to be surgically repaired. Sometimes a cleft palate is associated with a hare lip. This will be obvious to the doctor when she looks at the baby, and the parent can be reassured that this can be repaired surgically.
- Skin colour is observed. The baby should be pink, but occasionally she will appear to have slightly blue hands and feet, particularly if examined very soon after birth. She will usually 'pink up' quite quickly. A baby who is blue around the mouth and lips will need urgent medical care, as this is an indication that the heart and lungs are not functioning properly.
- Skin texture is noted. A premature baby may be covered with vernix (a greasy, protective covering over the skin) whereas a post mature baby may be born with dry flaky skin.
- Pigmentation and birth marks are also noted. Children with black skin sometimes have Mongolian blue spots (patches of darker skin that have the appearance of bruises) which are found particularly on the baby's bottom or back. Birth marks will generally fade with time.
- The hips are checked. Some children are born with a congenital dislocation of the hips and these babies will be referred to an orthopaedic surgeon for treatment.
- The doctor will listen to the baby's heart using a stethoscope to ascertain its rhythm and heart sounds. Any abnormalities may suggest congenital heart disease. Blue discoloration of the lips (cyanosis) is associated with some of the serious forms of congenital heart disease. Whilst listening to the heart, the doctor will check that the femoral pulses (pulses found in the groin) can be felt, as they can be very difficult to feel in a certain form of congenital heart disease.
- The doctor checks that the chest rises and falls symmetrically with each breath. She will also listen to the chest with a stethoscope to check there is air entry into both lungs.
- The spine is checked for evidence of spina bifida. This is a condition where one or two of the vertebra (the bones of the spine) have not completely fused together. Children born with evidence of spina bifida will be referred to a surgeon as a matter of some urgency. The spine is also checked for position: it should run down the centre of the back. Any curvature to one side (scoliosis) will need further investigation.

- The baby's muscle tone is also assessed. A baby who feels floppy may have cerebral palsy or Down's syndrome.
- The anus is checked for patency (whether it is open or not). This is done when the midwife checks the baby's rectal temperature soon after birth. The midwife will also note when the baby passes meconium (the first stool which is black and tarry) as this also confirms a patent anus.
- In a boy the testes are felt to determine whether or not they have descended into the scrotal sac. Undescended testes will usually descend within the first years of life. However, if they do not, surgical intervention will take place, usually before the child starts school. If left undescended, the child may be sterile when he is older, or, in some cases, undescended testes may undergo malignant change.

  The opening of the urethra is also checked; it should be at the end of the penis. Occasionally it opens on to one side of the penis (hypospadia) and surgical intervention may be required.
- In girls the labia are looked at. Occasionally they are fused together and may require surgery.
- The rectal temperature is taken, as it reflects as near to the central core temperature as possible. It is important to record the temperature soon after birth as the baby has been delivered from a temperature of 37°C (in the uterus) to a temperature of approximately 22°C in the delivery suite. A newborn baby has a poorly developed temperature regulating system and a large surface area from which to lose heat and is therefore prone to heat loss and the risk of hypothermia.
- The umbilical cord is checked to ensure that three blood vessels are present (there should be two arteries and one vein).
- The abdomen is checked for hernias. A hernia is a protrusion of a part of the bowel through a weakness in the abdominal wall. Babies with hernias will be referred to a surgeon. Hernias may be retractable (that is they will go back into the abdomen when gentle pressure is placed on them) or non-retractable in which case they will require urgent surgical intervention.
- Limbs should be symmetrical. Some babies are born with deformities of the lower limbs; the most common of these is talipes, a condition where the foot is not in correct alignment with the leg. These babies will be referred to the orthopaedic surgeon. The hands are checked for palmar creases – two are usually present. In a baby with Down's syndrome, only one palmar crease is seen. The number of digits are counted, extra digits are usually removed surgically.
- Reflex reactions are observed and Figure 7 should serve to remind the reader of the reflex reactions seen in the newborn.

Rooting reflex	The baby's cheek is touched; she will turn the head to locate with the mouth whatever has touched the cheek	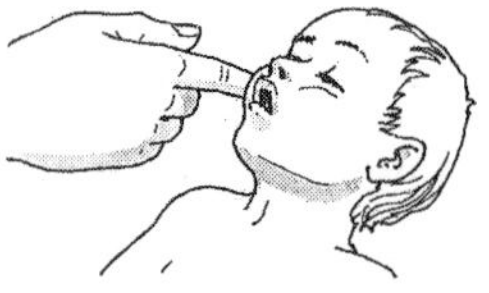
Grasp reflex	The baby will grasp anything put into her hand	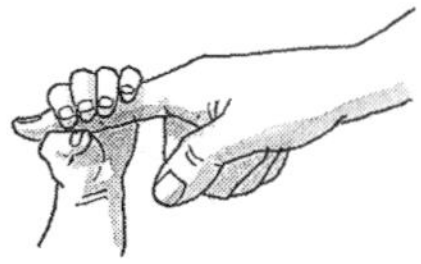
Stepping reflex	The baby is held up with one foot in contact with a surface. The other foot is brought up as though walking	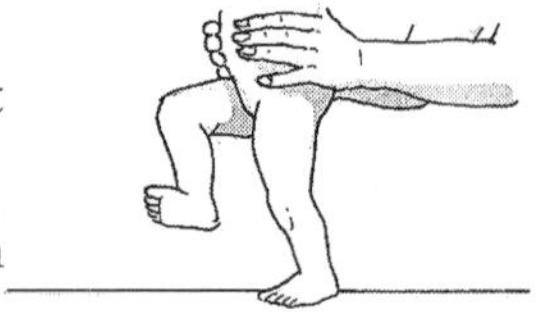
Sucking reflex	The baby will suck on anything put into her mouth	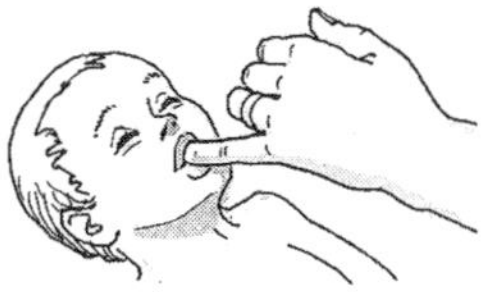
Moro (or startle) reflex	The baby will fling out the arms when startled. The hands are spread out and then clenched	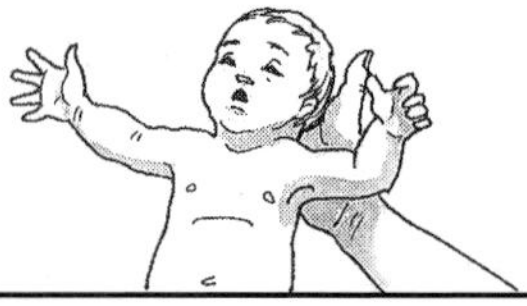

Figure 7 Babies are capable of a number of reflex actions

- **It is often difficult to ascertain whether or not a baby has any hearing loss.**
- **The baby's eyes are checked; the pupils should be of equal size and should constrict when a light is shone on them. The doctor will reflect a light off the back of the eye; the presence of a red reflex will exclude congenital cataract (an opacity of the lens that prevents the light reaching the back of the eye) and a rare but serious condition called retinoblastoma (a tumour of the retina).**

This concludes the examination at birth. The doctor will have written up her findings in the notes and if she is concerned about any finding she will arrange for the baby to be reviewed either urgently or routinely by a specialist or the baby's general practitioner. The midwife will do a blood test (the Guthrie test) by pricking the heel of the baby, on the seventh day after birth. This blood sample is sent to the laboratory to be analysed for evidence of phenylketonuria (see page 99) or hypothyroidism (see page 102).

The community midwife will visit the baby at home daily until the tenth day after birth. During this post natal period the general practitioner may also visit. The health visitor will visit ten to fourteen days after the birth to give advice on any problems, on general care and information about the child surveillance clinics.

The six-to-eight week check

Research has shown that the examinations at birth and at six-to-eight weeks show more abnormalities than any other routine early years examinations. Abnormalities that have developed since birth or that were not obvious at birth may now be detected. Any findings will be discussed with the parents and support will be offered if necessary. If any abnormalities are detected the baby will either be monitored at regular intervals or referred to a specialist.

The doctor or health visitor will often ask the parents if they have had any problems or concerns. These introductory remarks may lead to discussion on anything that is worrying them. Specifically, the doctor may ask about the baby's hearing and sight.

Whilst the doctor is waiting for the parent to undress the baby, she will observe the reactions of the baby and the mother, looking for smiles of enjoyment, eye contact and the ease with which the process is carried out, which can all serve as indicators of parental confidence.

PHYSICAL DEVELOPMENT

This examination follows a similar pattern to the examination at birth. In addition, the following points are noted and recorded:

- *General appearance.* This gives an indication of the general health and nourishment of the baby.
- *Weight.* The baby will be weighed naked and the weight will be plotted on a growth (centile) chart (see page 92).
- *Head circumference.* This will be measured and plotted on a growth chart (see page 95).
- *Posterior fontanelle.* This is usually closed by this time.
- *Head lag.* At birth the baby is unable to lift her head and if she is pulled up gently to a sitting position head lag is apparent (see Figure 8 on page 32). By the six-to-eight week check the head lag is still present, although it is not so pronounced.
- *When placed prone.* The baby will usually turn her head to one side.
- *Thumbs.* These are still held inwards with the fingers wrapped tightly around them.

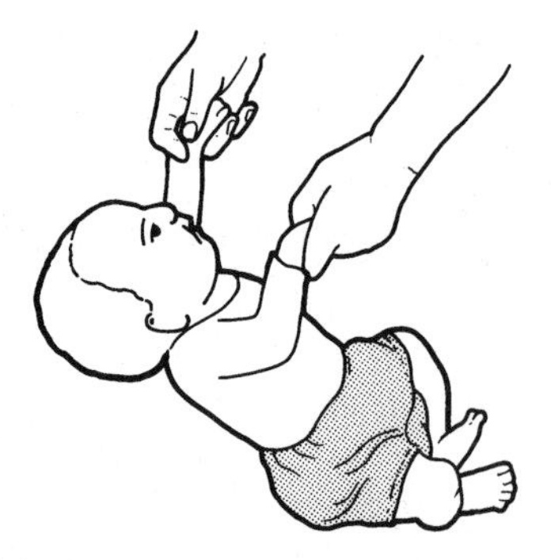

Figure 8 Head lag is apparent if the baby is pulled up

HEARING AND LANGUAGE

The parents will be asked if they think the baby can hear. A baby who can hear will 'startle' to a sudden noise.

At around this age the baby may make 'cooing' sounds and 'freeze' for some sounds.

VISION

The parents will be asked if they think the baby can see. The baby will usually turn her head to follow the mother. She will gaze intently into the face of the person who feeds her and will appear to be studying the face (see Figure 9). The baby's pupils will constrict when a bright light is shone into them.

SOCIAL

The baby is more responsive than when newly born. The feeding pattern is usually more predictable. If the baby is crying she will usually stop when picked up and will look at the person with great interest. By six weeks the baby will be smiling.

At the end of the examination the doctor will ensure that the Personal Child Health Record book is completed and will discuss her findings with the parents.

The examination at six-to-nine months

The doctor or health visitor will examine the baby and will observe the baby's interaction with the carer. Around this age the baby may be very clingy: this is to be expected. This examination may therefore take a little longer than previous examinations.

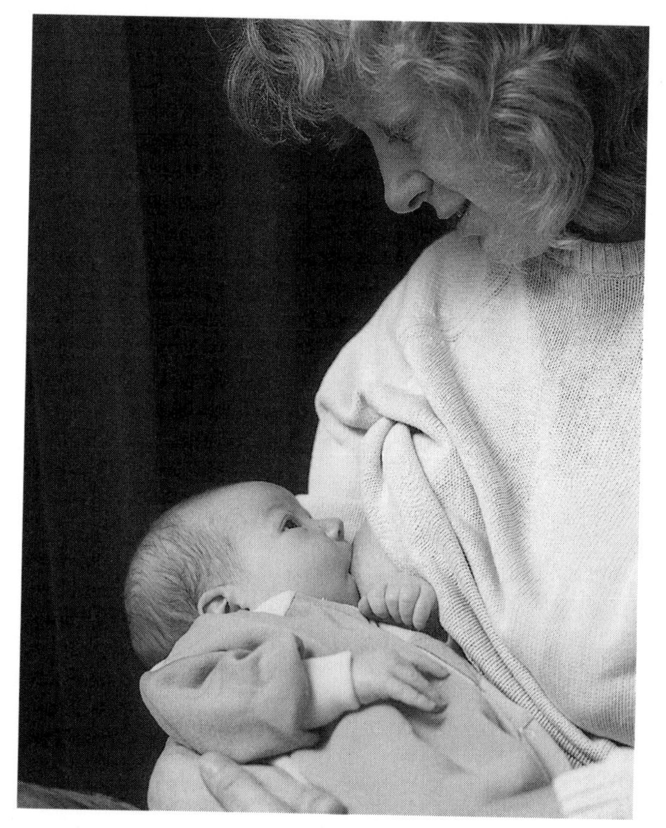

Figure 9 A baby will gaze intently at the person feeding her

PHYSICAL DEVELOPMENT

This examination follows a similar pattern to previous examinations. The following points are particularly noted and recorded:

- *Weight and head circumference.* These are measured and the results are plotted on the growth chart.
- *Sitting and rolling.* The parent is asked if the baby can perform these tasks, which are generally within the capabilities of a baby of this age.
- *Muscle tone.* This is observed, particularly when the baby is sitting on the carer's lap.
- *Grasping.* The baby is offered a toy which is usually taken with one hand and then passed to the other. The baby is observed for equal use of both hands and accuracy of grasping and passing.
- *Pincer grasp.* Some babies can, by this age, pick up hundreds and thousands using a pincer grasp. The hundreds and thousands are usually taken straight to the mouth where they can be safely eaten.

HEARING AND LANGUAGE

It is very important that any hearing loss is detected early, because it can lead to language and learning difficulties. It may be that the carer has detected a problem but as this is not always the case, all children are screened using a distraction test at this clinic.

Distraction test

This is carried out in a quiet room. Two people, one of whom is usually a health visitor, are present.

The aim of the test is to see if the child hears varying sound and pitch. The baby sits on the carer's lap. The helper sits in front of the baby and presents a distraction in the form of some sort of noiseless toy, thus gaining the baby's attention. The health visitor is positioned one metre behind the carer and child at an angle of 45°.

Once the 'distractor' has gained the baby's attention the distraction is minimised and the health visitor produces a sound. The child will turn her head in the direction of the sound if she hears it and this is taken to be a positive response. The process is repeated, this time with the health visitor being positioned one metre behind the baby at an angle of 45° from the

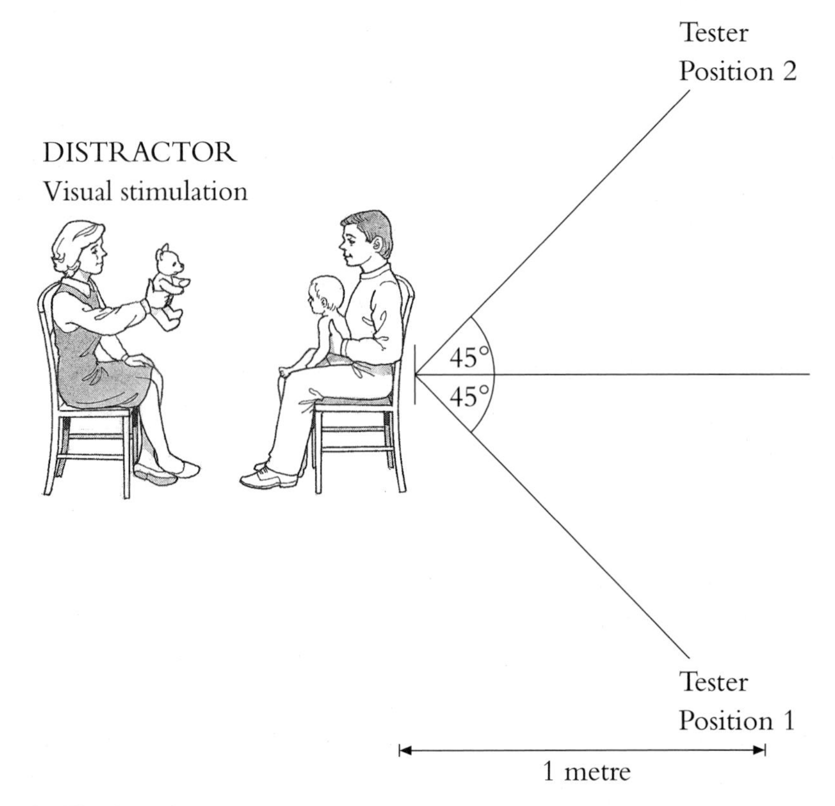

Figure 10 The distraction test

other ear. This process is repeated a number of times using sounds of varying frequency and pitch.

If a baby does not turn her head to a sound, it is repeated and if she still does not react it is taken that she has not heard the sound. If this happens for all or part of this hearing test, the health visitor will arrange to re-test the baby approximately one month later.

Babies may fail the distraction test for several reasons. It may be that the baby has a cold or an ear infection which affects hearing on a temporary basis. If she fails a second time the health visitor will refer the baby to an audiologist (hearing specialist).

The carer will be asked if the baby makes any sounds. She is usually 'cooing' at this stage and often chattering tunefully using consonant sounds. She may shout to gain attention and will listen and then shout again. The baby is often able to recognise voices, particularly her parents', will often listen when spoken to and may even try to carry on the 'conversation'.

Deaf children do vocalise but the vocalisations remain at a basic level. A baby who has not developed tuneful vocalisations by the age of eight months will usually be investigated for possible deafness.

A baby or child who has undetected hearing loss may show behavioural problems, which usually disappear quickly once the hearing loss has been corrected.

Vision

Whilst the child is playing, visual behaviour will be observed and she will be checked for signs of a squint which, if present, will require referral to an ophthalmologist (eye specialist).

Social

The baby is usually able to feed herself with some finger food and will try to grasp the spoon when being fed. She will be able to hold the bottle or feeding beaker and may even be able to take a drink successfully.

She takes part in games such as peek-a-boo and will imitate waving and hand clapping. At this stage she can distinguish strangers from those who are close to her and may demonstrate separation anxiety.

The two-year check

This follows the general pattern of the previous tests. The carer will be asked some questions about the baby's health in general. Any worries will be discussed.

PHYSICAL DEVELOPMENT

This follows the lines of the previous examinations:

- *General appearance.* This will give some indication of the general care and nourishment of the child.
- *Weight.* The child will be weighed and the weight will be plotted on a growth (centile) chart.
- *Height.* The child will be measured and the height will be plotted on the growth chart.
- *Head circumference.* This will be measured and plotted on a growth chart.
- *Walking.* At this stage the child is usually walking with a normal gait (manner of walking), can often manage stairs holding on to the rail and putting two feet to a step, and can run and use push-and-pull toys.
- *Manipulation.* The child can usually build a tower of six or seven bricks, can hold a pencil using thumb and two fingers and can turn the pages of a book one at a time.
- *Testes.* The carer will be asked if the testes are in the scrotal sac. If they are not the doctor will examine the child and refer him to a paediatric surgeon for an opinion as undescended testes are usually operated on before the child starts school.

HEARING AND LANGUAGE

The carer will be asked if there are any concerns about the child's hearing. If there are any worries the child will be referred to an audiologist for a hearing test and any treatment considered to be necessary.

The carer will be asked about the child's speech. A vocabulary of approximately 200 understandable words is common at this age. The child is usually able to string two or three words together and is continually asking questions.

SOCIAL

- *Potty training.* This is usually underway at this stage. Some children are clean and dry by day and in nappies at night, a few will be clean and dry at night, and some will still be in nappies. The health visitor is usually willing to discuss training and will give help and guidance as necessary.

- *Temper tantrums.* The child may throw temper tantrums when frustrated. These can sometimes be distressing for the carers and health visitors are willing to discuss the problems and offer advice.
- *Play.* The child will probably play near other children but not with them yet and will play alone in the vicinity of a carer.

The four-year check

The aim of this check is to detect any problems that might interfere with the child's education. As with all other checks, the parent is asked if they have any concerns about the child and in particular if there are any problems that might affect schooling.

PHYSICAL DEVELOPMENT

- *Weight.* The child will be weighed and the weight will be plotted on a growth (centile) chart.
- *Height.* The child will be measured and the height will be plotted on the growth chart.
- *Walking.* The carer will be asked specifically about walking. A child of this age can usually walk up and down stairs using one foot per stair, walk on tiptoe, hop and stand on one foot, then the other.
- *Manipulation.* The child usually has control of pencils and can draw and colour pictures.

Other checks will probably depend on concerns the carer or doctor may have, for instance, if the child has asthma an examination of the lungs may take place.

HEARING AND LANGUAGE

If the carer has any worries about hearing or sight the child is referred to an appropriate specialist.

The child can usually speak fairly fluently and enjoys reciting action rhymes (see Figure 11). He may be asked to name objects pictured on a language board.

SOCIAL

The child is more independent and can usually dress and undress with minimal assistance, use a knife and fork and wash her own hands and face.

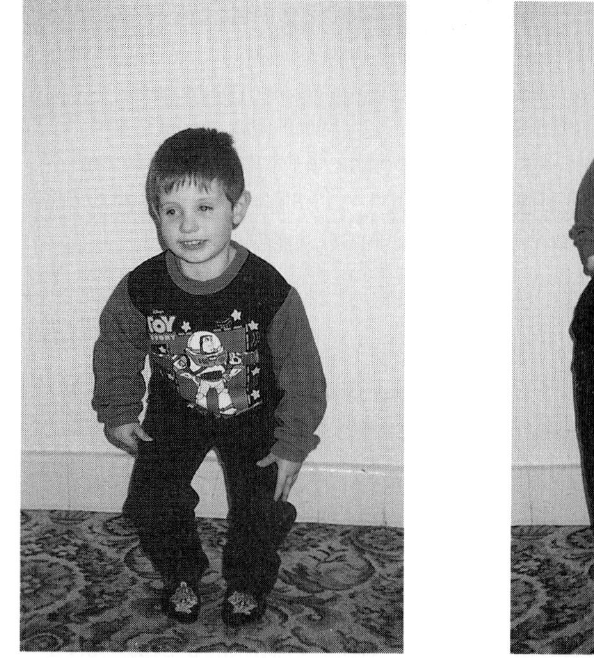

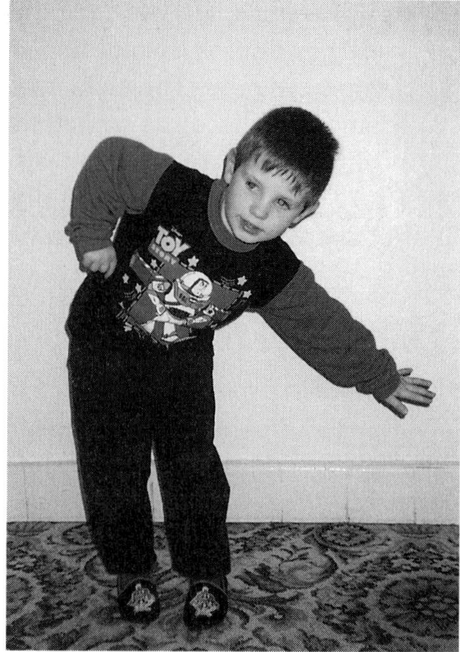

Figure 11 By four years, a child will be able to recite an action rhyme

Potty training is now generally complete and the child is clean and dry day and night, however some children continue to have the occasional accident at night.

Friendships may have often been formed and the child plays with friends, as opposed to alongside friends, at this stage.

Health promotion

All clinic visits provide an opportunity for health topics to be discussed. Any member of the primary health care team may be involved in making the most of these opportunities and topics include:

- prevention of accidents and safety issues
- weaning and nutrition
- dental care
- sun safety
- smoking and its adverse effects on the child.

ACTIVITY

Introduce yourself to a health visitor and ask permission to observe at a child health clinic. Aim to observe at least one health check at each age. Remember the importance of confidentiality. Keep a record of what you learn from your observations.

ACTIVITY

Working in a small group, take one of the health promotion topics from the list above. Research the topic and devise a plan to present the information to a small group of parents or carers in a clinic setting.

You should aim to discuss the topic for no more than ten minutes, but think about planning a display in the waiting room to back up your information. You should also contact your nearest health promotion unit and request leaflets that are relevant to your topic so that you can give these to the parents or early years workers to remind them of the information you discussed with them. You will also need to consider where they might be able to acquire further information.

Conclusion

Child health clinics provide an opportunity for health promotion, the early detection of abnormalities and support for parents and carers in a social setting. As a result of their training and experience, child carers can make valuable contributions to the development of children in their care. The informal setting of the clinics encourages carers to discuss worries or anxieties they might otherwise feel reluctant to mention.

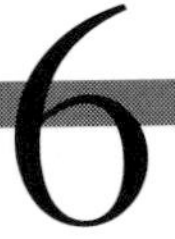

Recognising the Ill Child

Adults tend to tell everyone if they are feeling unwell. This is really a request for sympathy and tolerance; it is also a warning signal that they might be less efficient and tolerant than usual. Young children have neither the knowledge from past experiences to interpret what they are feeling nor the communication skills to express any warnings. Carers therefore need to be able to identify and interpret any warning signals. The professional carer should as part of her training become well practised in the art of observation. This skill serves as a good grounding for child care, enabling her to be sensitive to children's needs.

Possible clues that the child is ill

This section will serve as a guide to possible clues but as all children are individuals it is very important that the carer 'tunes in' to her own charges, interpreting their individual signals.

Changes in behaviour

Behavioural changes may be apparent when children are unwell. They may be quieter than usual, more clingy, appear to be attention seeking or perhaps whining or irritable. The sleep pattern may alter, with some children sleeping more than usual and some sleeping less. Children may be less energetic or appear to regress (behave as if they are younger).

Some children may show less interest in their toys or choose toys that they have previously outgrown. Ill children like to watch television or videos as this activity requires less effort than playing.

Carers need to remind themselves that these features are related to the child's inability to express the problem vocally. One or several of these features will often precede an illness. It must be remembered that there is no time limit on these changes; sometimes they may be apparent for only a few hours, while at other times they may continue for a few days.

Communication

Carers become experts at 'reading' **non-verbal** cues, the body language that is an important part of successful caring for children. When caring for ill children it is even more important to interpret the non-verbal cues as these might enable them to assess the nature and urgency of the illness. Facial expression can, for instance, show pain but sometimes assessing the severity of the pain may be difficult. Non-verbal cues can be good indicators of the problem. A look at the child's face, the position she has adopted and movement (which may be limited) may, for instance, give a clear indication of a broken bone.

Crying is a sign of distress, perhaps caused by pain or fear. Babies may cry more than usual when they are unwell. Sometimes it is possible to detect different types of cries in babies, for example, those of pain or hunger. A shrill high-pitched cry associated with other signs and symptoms may indicate meningitis. A whimpering cry may indicate exhaustion. Older children will sometimes cry but not yet have the linguistic abilities to explain the reason.

Verbal cues may or may not be reliable. The ability to use language successfully will depend on the child's age, stage of development and to some extent on past experiences. A four-year-old may complain of a headache at the same time as clutching her tummy. Young children may give unreliable answers to closed questions as they often tend to answer 'yes' to whatever they are asked.

Physical signs

Skin

Ill children often have a pale appearance, but if they have a raised temperature the face may be flushed. If there is severe difficulty in breathing they may appear blue at the extremities such as the fingernails, or have a blue appearance centrally, for example inside the lips (which are usually pink in all people regardless of ethnic origin). Note: if a child is blue either at the extremities or centrally a doctor should be called urgently (see page 47). A yellow tinge may be seen in children who have jaundice and this is most noticeable in the white of the eye (the sclera) or under the tongue.

Skin rashes may be seen in some infectious and allergic conditions. The distribution and colour will vary according to the cause. Whilst there are lots of different types of rashes – these are described in more detail under the

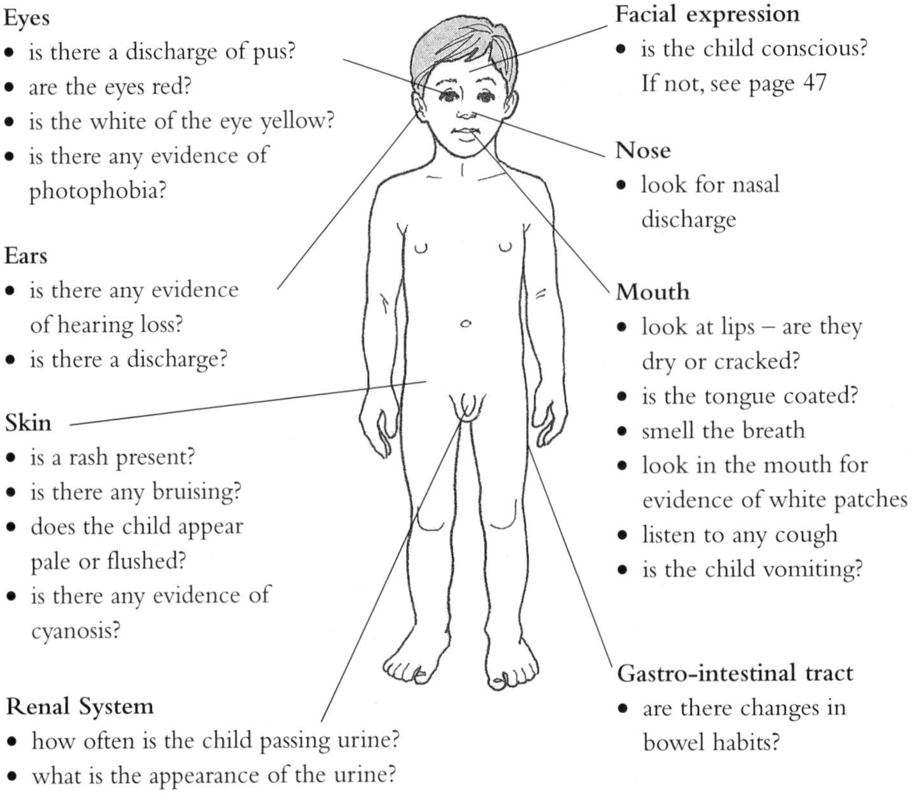

Eyes
- is there a discharge of pus?
- are the eyes red?
- is the white of the eye yellow?
- is there any evidence of photophobia?

Ears
- is there any evidence of hearing loss?
- is there a discharge?

Skin
- is a rash present?
- is there any bruising?
- does the child appear pale or flushed?
- is there any evidence of cyanosis?

Renal System
- how often is the child passing urine?
- what is the appearance of the urine?

Facial expression
- is the child conscious? If not, see page 47

Nose
- look for nasal discharge

Mouth
- look at lips – are they dry or cracked?
- is the tongue coated?
- smell the breath
- look in the mouth for evidence of white patches
- listen to any cough
- is the child vomiting?

Gastro-intestinal tract
- are there changes in bowel habits?

Figure 12 Possible physical signs of illness

specific conditions – many are seen for only a short time. Bruising is often seen in young children and is partly due to the nature of their unsteadiness. It is commonly seen on the shins. However, excessive bruising, particularly in unusual places such as the trunk, bottom and back may suggest an illness such as leukaemia, or child abuse. Note: a Mongolian blue spot may be mistaken for a bruise; these are blue/grey patches seen on the lower back or buttocks of Asian or black babies, they usually disappear by the age of four or five. Skin will lose its elasticity when a child becomes dehydrated.

Expression

The expression may indicate discomfort or pain.

Mouth

Dry or cracked lips may occur, for instance, if the child has been mouth breathing. The tongue may be coated; this is usually a non-specific sign as it may occur in a variety of conditions. The breath may smell; this may be a non-specific sign but it is particularly noticeable with some infections, for example tonsillitis. A sweet-smelling breath characteristically described as smelling of pear drops may occur in diabetes. The mucous membrane inside the mouth may have white patches on it and the gums may show evidence of infection, that is swelling or even pus.

Nose

There may be a nasal discharge, the quantity and colour of which should be noted, for example thick and green or clear and bloody.

Eyes

An eye infection may lead to a discharge of pus and this may be thick enough to result in the child being unable to open her eyes after a sleep (see Chapter 12). The eyes may appear red if the temperature is raised or if an eye infection is present. A yellow tinge in the sclera is seen in the child with jaundice. There may be signs caused by the child rubbing the eyes due to crying or itching. Photophobia (the dislike of light) may be apparent if the child turns away when placed near a bright window or if she protests when the light is turned on. This may be an important sign in meningitis.

Ears

There may be intermittent or permanent hearing loss. A child who rubs or frequently touches her ear(s) may be in pain. A discharge of pus, which is often smelly, may be apparent with some ear infections. After a head injury there may be a straw-coloured discharge from either the ear or nose, indicating loss of cerebro-spinal fluid. Note: if this is seen medical assistance should be urgently sought.

Respiratory Tract

A child's cough may be described as wheezy (a characteristic high-pitched whistling sound heard when the child breathes out), productive (when the child coughs up phlegm (sputum) which is usually swallowed), dry (non-productive), barking or whooping (a characteristic sound made when the child breathes in) depending on the underlying cause of the cough. If the child makes a grunting noise when attempting to cough and particularly if there is evidence of rib recession (the ribs appearing to be sucked in) an urgent request for medical help should be made, as this could be an indication of respiratory obstruction.

Coughs are nearly always worse at night and some but not all children are distressed by the situation. The respiratory rate may increase, for instance, if the child has pneumonia.

Renal System

The child may pass urine more frequently than usual, or it may be painful to pass urine, if there is a urinary tract infection, in which case the urine may smell or appear cloudy. If dehydrated, little urine will be passed, and it will appear dark with a 'strong' smell. If a baby has more than one dry nappy over a period of several hours, medical advice should be sought. The previously potty-trained child may be incontinent more often than would usually be accepted as the 'odd accident'.

Gastro-intestinal System

Children have a decreased appetite and are fussier about their food when unwell. Changes in bowel habit may be apparent, with the child developing constipation or diarrhoea. Vomiting may be associated with many conditions and the content, frequency and nature of the vomiting (for instance, is it projectile?) should be noted. Any blood in the vomit or stools should be reported to the doctor.

Nervous System

The conscious level may alter in some circumstances, for example, after a head injury, when medical help should be urgently requested. The following terms refer to levels of consciousness: fully conscious – alert and responsive; unconscious – unaware of surroundings and not rousable. Between these levels there are degrees of consciousness referring to, for instance, unusual drowsiness and slurred speech.

Cardiac system

The heart rate may increase particularly if there is evidence of a raised temperature. This may be felt as an increased pulse rate. A hypothermic (body temperature below 35°C) child, on the other hand, will have a slow heart rate.

Temperature (also see page 60)

A child may develop a high temperature as a result of an infection. The child may appear flushed and feel hot, thirsty and irritable. If the temperature becomes very high she may hallucinate and become very agitated. There is a possibility that a febrile convulsion may occur.

A hypothermic child, on the other hand, may be cold to the touch and have a flushed face despite the cold temperature, and appear to be immobile and have shallow breathing.

Note: These signs and symptoms tend to build up gradually over several hours or even days. However, in some circumstances they may appear acutely. The carer should make a careful note of the signs and symptoms as these will be discussed if the child is taken to see the doctor.

When to seek medical advice

It is difficult to give a definitive list of all occasions when medical advice should be sought. The carer will, of course, need to use their own judgement remembering that they know the child best and can pick up even the most subtle changes which may indicate that the child is unwell. If the carer is worried about the health of any child in her care, medical advice should be sought from the GP or health visitor, who will be happy to give telephone advice. *If in doubt seek reassurance.*

Medical advice should be sought in the following circumstances.

Crying

If the child:

- cries for an unusually long time and is inconsolable
- is crying differently from usual, for instance a baby or child may whimper when very unwell
- cries and has other associated signs.

Feeding

If the child:

- will not feed or suck
- refuses food or drinks (particularly drinks) over an unusually long period of time.

Vomiting

If the child:

- vomits for more than six hours
- vomits and appears to be in pain or dehydrated
- vomits after a head injury.

Change in bowel habits

If the child:

- has frequent loose stools

- passes blood in the stools
- is constipated, particularly if it is associated with discomfort when passing stools.

Breathing difficulties

If the child:

- has any difficulty breathing, for example wheezing
- is choking (an ambulance should be called if first-aid measures are ineffective)
- has a barking cough
- cannot breathe freely
- is too breathless to talk
- has rib recession (appears to be sucking in the muscles between the ribs) and difficulty in breathing
- complains of pain on breathing
- coughs up blood.

Temperature (see page 60)

If the child:

- has a raised temperature and other signs of illness
- feels hot and appears to have neck stiffness and/or dislike of light
- has a raised temperature and a fit (febrile convulsion)
- feels cold and is listless.

Conscious level

If the child:

- has recently sustained a head injury and feels sick or vomits, or there is a change in conscious level; or if the pupils are no longer equal in size
- has a change in conscious level without any of the above signs
- is drowsy and difficult to rouse and/or does not recognise people
- is unusually quiet or listless.

Pain

If the child:

- has a suspected fracture
- appears to be in pain
- is unable to use any part of her body.

Emergency situations

In an emergency call an ambulance immediately. If possible also call the doctor, as she may arrive before the ambulance, will probably know the child's history and be able to initiate treatment. The child should not be given anything to eat or drink until seen by the doctor.

Emergencies are when the child:

- stops breathing
- is having difficulty breathing and is going blue (or may appear 'waxy')
- is unconscious
- is bleeding and it cannot be controlled
- has eaten or drunk any toxic substance, such as bleach
- has sustained a serious burn
- has a chemical in the eye
- is in any situation where life is at risk.

The early years worker's role when a child is unwell

1 Inform the next-of-kin. It is imperative that a contact number is kept to hand. If there is an emergency the next-of-kin should be contacted as soon as possible after the emergency has been dealt with.

2 On the instructions of the next-of-kin, arrange for a doctor to see the child. This will involve telephoning the surgery to request an appointment.

While the child is being examined the early years worker should:

3 Stay with the child at all times. This is reassuring to the child and allows the early years worker to assist if necessary.

4 Prepare the child as much as possible. Remember the child is feeling unwell and may be irritable and frightened. When talking to the child use language that she understands and be patient in your explanations.

5 Assist the doctor as necessary.

6 Undress the child, as appropriate. Remember to ask their permission.

7 Give the history of the illness to the doctor clearly and concisely. Be accurate in the description, include your observations and any other information thought necessary. Do not be afraid to offer an opinion, for example, 'I have noticed that she has pulled at her ear in the last few hours. Perhaps it is painful?' Do not be afraid to clarify points.

8 Include relevant past medical history including any allergic reactions, particularly if the doctor is not the child's usual doctor.

9 When the examination is over the doctor will give some explanation and probably some instructions. Clarify the information and write it down if necessary (remember, you will need to relay the information to the parents). The following information will be needed: the diagnosis (what is wrong with the child); the treatment; additional instructions; the reaction of the child; any follow-up information; and the date and time of any further appointment.

10 Take the child home, unless an admission to hospital is necessary. Reassure the child. Allow her plenty of time to rest and follow the instructions given.

Examination of the child

The examination will depend to some extent on the history given and may involve some of the following:

- The child's temperature may be taken.
- Palpation for swollen glands. Lymph glands may swell when there is an infection; their detection will help in the diagnosis (see Figure 13).
- An examination of the ear may take place. The child will be shown the auroscope and positioned as shown in Figure 14, page 50. This will enable the doctor to examine her as quickly as possible and with the minimum distress.
- An examination of the eye will involve a general observation of the inflammation and infection (as in conjunctivitis), or a more detailed examination of the back of the eye using an ophthalmoscope or the installation of some drops to assist the examination.
- For an examination of the throat, position the child as shown in Figure 15, page 50. Young children find the examination of the throat slightly unpleasant, but a securely held child, held as shown in the diagram,

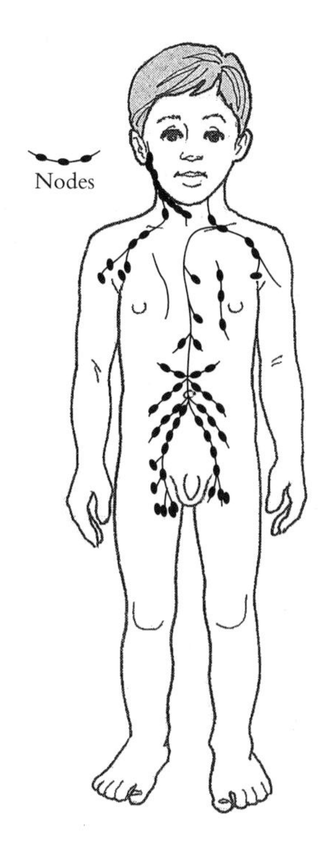

Figure 13 The lymphatic system

enables the doctor to get a good view of the throat and to complete the procedure as quickly as possible.

- During the examination the doctor will observe the skin for rashes, colour and general appearance. She may ask questions about any observations.
- It will be necessary to remove the child's outer clothing and lift their vest to examine the chest. A small child is usually examined sitting on the carer's lap. An older child will sit on a chair. The doctor will often let a small child play with the stethoscope before putting it on the chest so that she is familiar with it. During this time, the doctor will be noting the respiratory rate and observing the chest to check, for example, for rib recession. She will then listen to the front and the back of the chest for air entry into the lungs and then count the heart rate (see Figures 16 and 17, page 51).
- For the examination of the abdomen, a young baby may be more easily examined sitting on the carer's lap. An older child should lie on the bed or couch as shown in Figure 18, page 52.
- If meningitis is a possibility, the doctor may examine the child for neck stiffness. The child should be positioned on her back (see Figure 19, page 52).

(*Text continues on page 53*)

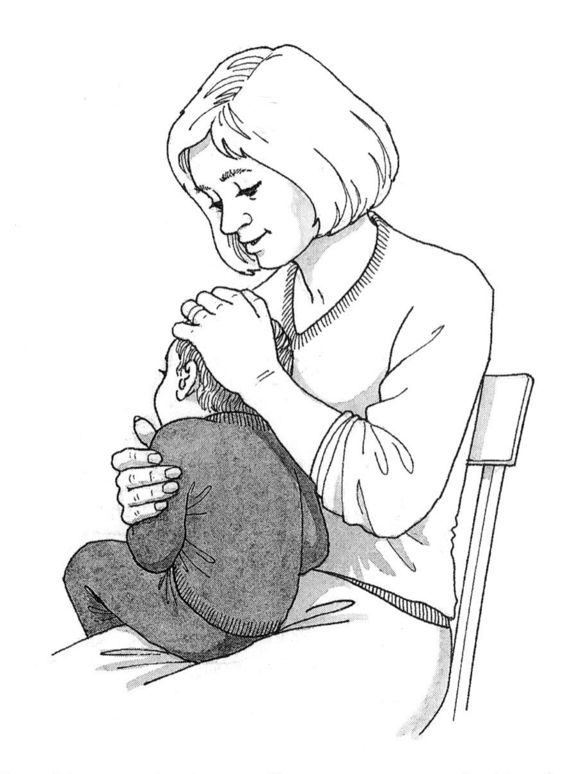

Figure 14 Examination of the ear – the doctor will use an auroscope. Position the child to one side, and make her comfortable. Hold both arms by the side and gently hold the head steady. After examination of one ear, turn the child the other way

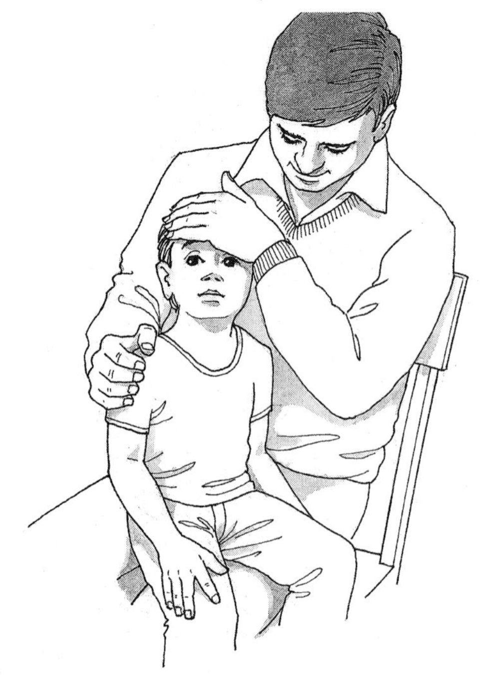

Figure 15 Examination of the throat – position the child facing the doctor. Gently restrain the arms at the sides and support the head. The doctor will ask the child to open the mouth and will then depress the tongue to gain a good view of the throat

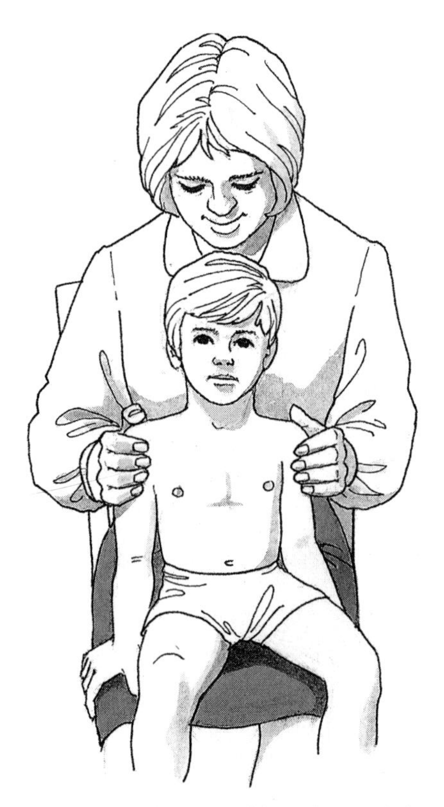

Figure 16 Examination of the chest – position the child on the carer's lap, facing the doctor. Hold the arms gently at the sides

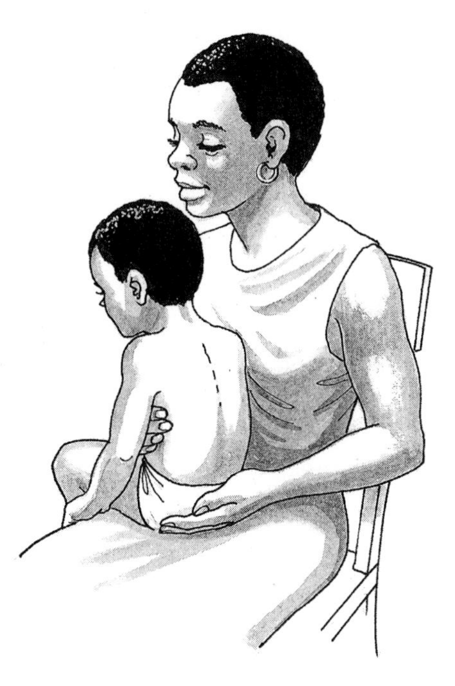

Figure 17 Examination of the chest – position the child to one side so that the doctor may listen to the back of the chest

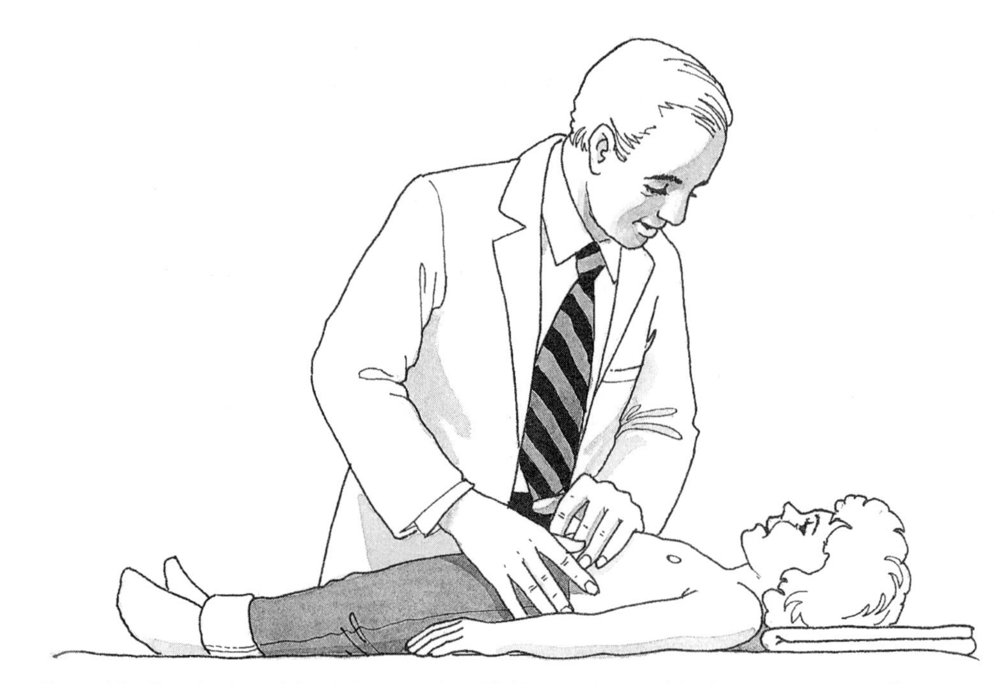

Figure 18 Examination of the abdomen – the child lies on the couch in the prone position. The carer should stay with the child to ensure safety and to reassure her

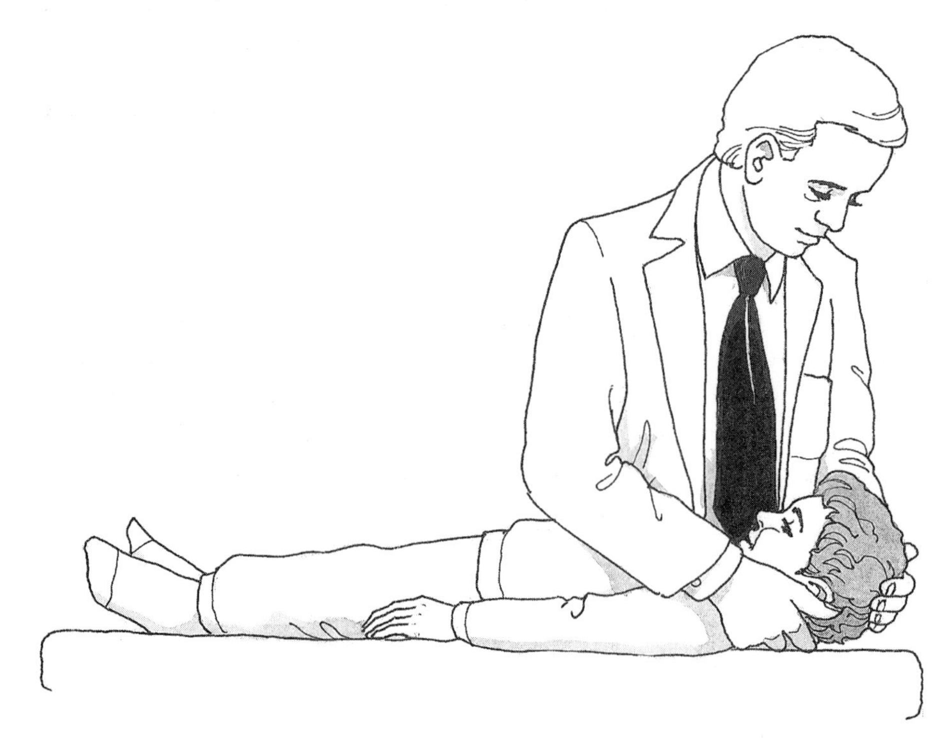

Figure 19 Examination of the neck for stiffness – the child lies prone without a pillow. The doctor will tell the child to relax while holding the head. The head will then be lifted up and forwards. A child with neck stiffness will resist this. The carer should stay near the child to ensure safety and to reassure her

- If a fracture or sprain is suspected, the doctor may look at the affected limb and then compare it with the other limb. Any swelling is then more obvious.

The examination may reveal that the child will need further investigation in which case she will be referred to a specialist as necessary.

ACTIVITY

Reflect on how you feel when you are unwell (most people have at least had a common cold and felt under the weather for a period of time). Write down your memories and then attempt to recall these when a child in your care is next unwell. Your reflections may help you to empathise with the child.

Does your behaviour change and, if so, in what ways?

Think about the verbal and non-verbal cues you communicate.

What happens to your colour and your appearance?

Write down the signs and symptoms you remember and then attempt to put yourself in the child's shoes and consider how it might feel if you could not fully communicate your feelings.

Conclusion

This chapter has taken the reader on a tour of possible clues that might suggest the child is unwell. A carer should seek medical advice at any time if she is worried, and a guide has been included to aid decision making if the carer is unsure whether to seek help or not. The examination of the child has been included to assist the carer when she takes the child to the doctor.

7

Principles of Caring for the Ill Child

Ill children require extra attention from the people they trust the most, their parents or regular carer. It is these people who can provide the understanding and patience necessary.

The needs of the ill child

Children react to illness in different ways, depending on many factors, such as age, stage of development, family expectations and previous experience of illness. Maslow's hierarchy of needs is a useful model on which to base the needs of children and adults (see Figure 20).

It is pictured as a triangle depicting the importance of attending to the physical needs before all others. This of course makes sense, because without food, water, warmth, shelter and clothing survival is impossible. Once these physical requirements have been met attention can be given to the safety

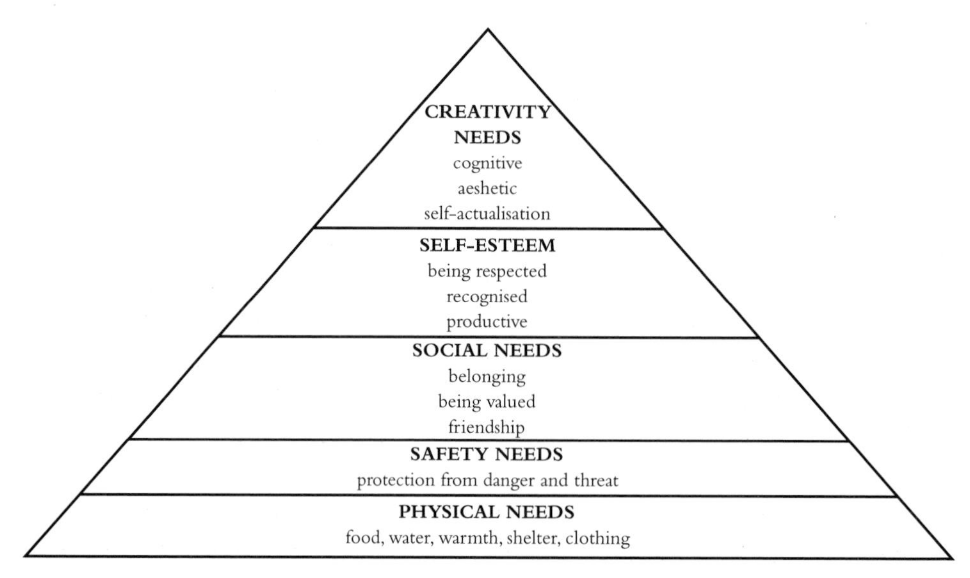

Figure 20 Maslow's hierarchy of needs

needs of providing protection so that the individual feels safe in her surroundings. The next layer relates to the social needs. These are concerned with the importance of belonging, of being loved and cared for by family and friends. Individuals of all ages need to feel recognised and respected. These needs are concerned with self-esteem and using Maslow's pyramid they can best be met once the social needs are in place. The final layer is concerned with creativity which incorporates cognitive (perception and problem solving) needs, aesthetic (appreciation and enjoyment of beautiful things) needs and self-actualisation (the need to function and reach full potential).

This pyramid of needs must be considered as a *continuous* process and as one need is met another takes its place. It is included here to serve as a model for the reader when caring for the sick child and provides a framework on which to meet the needs of each child. Using the model the layers of the pyramid will be considered in turn.

Physical needs

FOOD

A child's appetite decreases during illness, therefore small amounts of attractively presented food should be offered to encourage eating. Sometimes the child will refuse food in the short-term, that is for one or two days, and it is not necessarily cause for concern provided the child is drinking plenty of fluids.

Some conditions, such as cystic fibrosis or diabetes, require a special diet and a dietician will advise the parents accordingly and give advice to cover illness.

FLUIDS

A good fluid intake should be maintained when the child is unwell as it will help to reduce a raised temperature, and prevent dehydration. Children should be encouraged to drink plenty of fluids and if this proves difficult tempting them with fluids that are only offered on special occasions, such as Coca-Cola, might help. Ice lollies or ice pops are excellent particularly if the child has a raised temperature, as they have the added bonus of having a cooling effect. It must be remembered that children often regress when they are unwell, that is, they gain comfort from adopting comforts that they had previously discarded, for example, drinking from a bottle instead of a cup. This should not be discouraged as these habits may make the child feel more secure and when health is regained the child will revert to the more grown-up way of behaving.

ELIMINATION

Bowel habits often change during an illness, and medical advice may be necessary. Constipation may be avoided by ensuring the child has a good fluid intake and eats some fruit and vegetables. The urinary output may decrease as the body loses fluid if the temperature is raised. If the urinary output is very low then medical advice should be sought. In babies, this is indicated by dry nappies.

If the child is incontinent or has diarrhoea she will need to be reassured and the area should be washed and dried and a barrier cream used. Clean clothes (and if necessary clean bed linen) will be required.

FRESH AIR

Good ventilation is essential and the window may be opened to circulate fresh air.

WARMTH

Over-heating or under-heating can both have serious consequences. The room temperature for a newborn baby should be kept between 18°C and 21°C. As the child grows up the temperature regulating system becomes established and the room temperature can be decreased slightly.

Children should be clothed so that they feel comfortable in the surroundings. See Temperature Control at the end of this section.

HYGIENE

An ill child will feel more comfortable if washed regularly. A daily bath is not essential, although it may be enjoyed by many children. The child's hands, teeth, face and bottom area should be washed twice a day. Clothes and bedclothes will need to be changed and washed more frequently than usual. The carer must maintain a high standard of hygiene at all times to prevent additional illness.

Safety needs

Safety is of paramount importance and the carer needs to be conscientious in this respect.

- **It is important that she is vigilant for any change in the child's condition that might indicate that a medical opinion should be sought.**

- If the child is taking medication the carer should ensure that unwanted effects of the medication are known so that if the child develops any of these they can be reported to the doctor.
- If specialist equipment is necessary the carer should know how to use it safely.
- Some conditions, such as croup, get worse at night and ideally the child should be allowed to sleep in the same room as the parent so that a quick response can be made if necessary.

Medical Care

See 'When to seek medical advice' in Chapter 6, and Chapter 8 for advice on medication.

Medication must be given as directed. A knowledge of common unwanted effects should be known and if there is any evidence of unwanted effects they must be reported to the doctor.

If the child's condition deteriorates and the carer is worried about the child, a doctor should be consulted. If admission to hospital seems likely, the child should be prepared (see Chapter 15).

Comfort

Changes in the child's life, including illness, may lead to feelings of insecurity. Carers can help the child to overcome these feelings by showing understanding and sympathy. Reassurance and comfort help to provide security in times of stress and can be achieved by paying attention to several considerations.

Children like to be cared for in their own environment and when they are unwell they like a parent to be present (if this is not possible then a relative or a person who is well known to the child).

When children are unwell they tend to prefer to be near the family and not shut away in their own room. It is a relatively simple task to make up a bed for day time use in the main living room or even in the kitchen if that is where the family spends most of the time. In this way the carer can continue with the household chores when the child sleeps and is there for the child on waking.

Communicating with the child is important. Use language the child understands to interpret non-verbal cues, for instance, when helping her to describe the area affected by pain.

Regression is common in children when they are unwell. This should be accepted and is a form of comfort. The child will usually revert to her usual behaviour pattern on recovery.

The child will need more time and attention, as we all do when we are unwell. The carer will have to defer non-essential tasks until the child recovers.

Trust is built on telling the truth. The child will find it reassuring to be told she will soon be well again. If it is unlikely that health will be regained it is advisable to take advice from the professionals on how to approach this with the child.

Security objects such as 'cuddlies' or teddies are important if the child has one. Many children are very attached to these objects and they provide comfort.

If the child does need to be admitted to hospital then it is very comforting to her if a parent stays throughout the admission.

Social needs

SOCIAL CONTACT

When the child is unwell she will probably only want her parents or carers to be near. As the child improves, visits from friends or relatives are enjoyed, however, these may prove tiring and the carer may have to suggest a time limit. They may not be possible if the child's disease is infectious.

If the child is unwell for a long time and attends nursery, playgroup or school, the teacher may arrange for the other children to write and this may act as a morale booster.

CULTURAL DIFFERENCES

The early years worker will need to be familiar with any cultural differences which could affect the care of the child. Parents will usually give guidance on such issues.

Self-esteem needs

PLAY AND ACTIVITY

Play is an essential part of normal development for all children. During illness play can act as a distraction giving the child something to do and providing security for the child as it is an everyday activity. Regression should not be discouraged.

With a little forethought, imaginative play seen in well children can be continued. For instance, even the child who is bed bound can be involved in painting. Play also provides an opportunity for physiotherapy which may be part of the recovery process, for example, the child who has injured an arm could through play be encouraged to use the other arm. The physiotherapist may suggest particular play activities to encourage the use of certain muscles.

If the child has periods of feeling better and wants to play outside, this may be encouraged as long as the weather is suitable. It is important that she is dressed appropriately and supervised at all times. Note: Children with infectious diseases should not play with other children who have not had the disease.

Play provides an opportunity for the sick child to act out frustrations and anxieties caused by the illness. It is important for the development of good self-esteem and is as essential when the child is ill (during the periods of feeling better) as it is when the child is well. It allows them to be creative and develop their thinking processes, making sense of the situation.

ACTIVITY

Using the pyramid depicting Maslow's hierarchy of needs, write on the following:

- **How you would meet the needs of a two-year-old child who has been vomiting for four hours**
- **How you would meet the needs of a baby who has developed a cold and has a slightly raised temperature.**

ACTIVITY

You are working in a day nursery. The policy of the nursery is that children who are unwell should be taken home by a parent.

In pairs, role play the following scenario.

During the course of the morning, a four-year-old girl becomes uncharacteristically quiet and irritable. She is pale and refuses a mid-morning drink. As the morning progresses it becomes very obvious that she is unwell. The supervisor asks you to telephone her mother and request that the child be taken home.

You telephone the mother who is in an important meeting and she is 'not to be disturbed'. How will you tackle the situation? Develop this scenario using several outcomes.

Temperature

Body temperature

Normal body temperature is between 36 and 37°C (96.8–98.4°F). A body temperature over 37.5°C is called a fever or **pyrexia** (a 'temperature'). A body temperature of 35°C or less is called **hypothermia**. Remember that temperatures quoted are temperatures that have been taken orally (in the mouth); a temperature taken under the axilla (in the armpit) is slightly lower than an oral temperature (by approximately 0.5°C).

Body temperature does vary slightly throughout the day and is usually found to be slightly higher in the evening. If you suspect that a child in your care has a raised temperature, you should measure it. If a doctor's advice needs to be sought they may ask for the temperature reading and it is helpful to be specific.

A baby has an immature temperature-regulating centre in the brain. This, in part, explains why temperatures may fluctuate, with a baby 'burning up' one minute and the temperature only being slightly raised a little later.

Thermometers

There are several types of thermometers available; the traditional one is the mercury thermometer. Others include digital thermometers and the fever

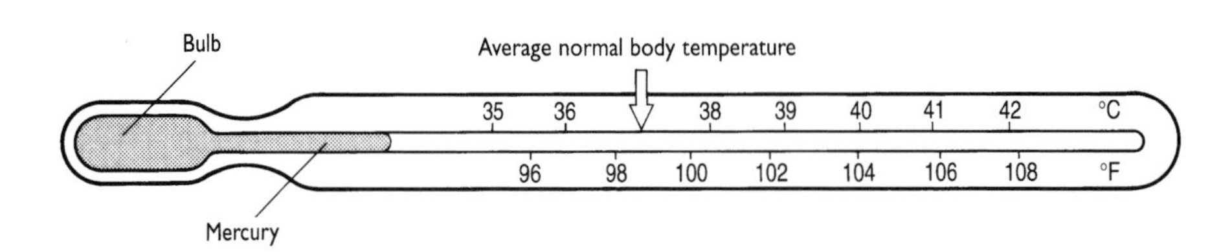

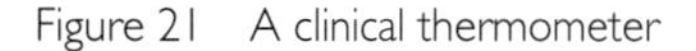
Figure 21 A clinical thermometer

strip (sometimes called the liquid crystal thermometer). The digital thermometer is slightly more expensive than a mercury thermometer, but has the advantage of being easily read and less hazardous because it is not made of glass and there is no mercury within it. The fever strip is easy to use but due to its lack of sensitivity it is not recommended. A new type of thermometer used in hospitals and some health centres fits into the ear and measures the temperature within thirty seconds.

Taking the child's temperature

In order to take the child's temperature the sequence below should be followed:

- Collect the equipment.
- Find books or toys to be used as distractions.
- Use language that the child will understand and tell her what you are going to do.
- Sit the child on your knee.

Using a digital thermometer under the arm:

- Take the thermometer out of the case.
- Place the thermometer under the arm as shown in Figure 22, page 62.
- The thermometer should be read when the temperature stops rising. Some digital thermometers will beep when this point is reached.

Using a mercury thermometer:

- Shake the mercury to the bottom of the thermometer.
- Place the thermometer under the child's arm.
- Hold the child as shown in Figure 22 thus protecting the thermometer from breaking.
- Read to the child or play in this limited position until the thermometer has finally measured the temperature (this may take up to five minutes).

Remember, never leave a child alone with a mercury thermometer – it is made of glass which could break and it contains mercury which, if exposed, poses a health hazard.

Hypothermia

Hypothermia describes the state when the body temperature drops below 35°C. Babies are prone to hypothermia for several reasons:

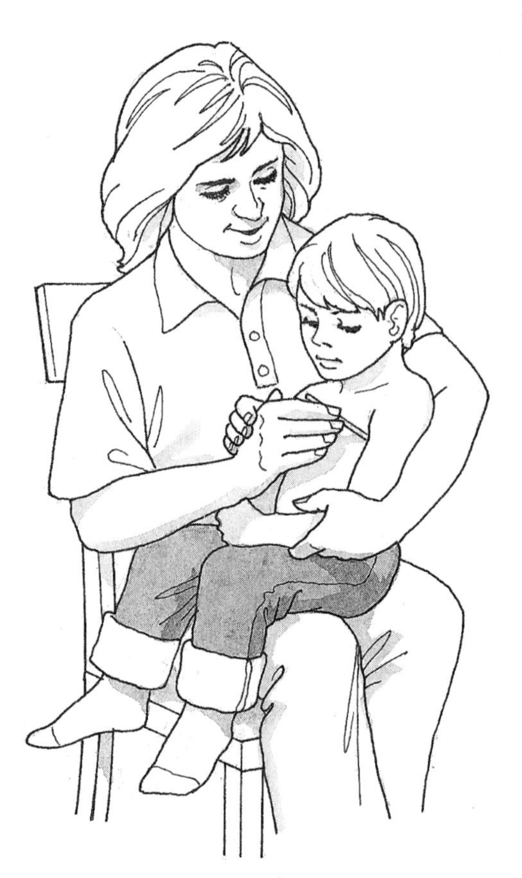

Figure 22 Taking the axillary temperature – the parent or carer sits with the child on the lap. A mercury thermometer is shaken until the mercury is below the reading of 35°C. A digital thermometer needs no preparation. The thermometer is placed under the child's arm and held there while the reading is taken. It may help to distract the child during this process

- They have a relatively large surface area from which to lose heat.
- They are unable to shiver, so they cannot regain body heat once it has been lost.
- They are relatively inactive and therefore depend on their carer to dress them adequately for their environment.
- Their temperature-regulating system is poorly developed.

Hypothermia may cause death. If the carer suspects that the baby or child may be hypothermic, a low-reading thermometer will need to be used. If one is not available there is no time for delay – medical help should be sought *immediately*.

How to Recognise a Hypothermic Child

- The child is cold to the touch. This is because the blood vessels to the skin have constricted in an attempt to conserve heat. This occurs because the body is trying to maintain a constant temperature to the major organs so that vital functions are maintained. If the carer suspects the child has hypothermia, a good indicator is to feel the child's abdomen or under the child's arm, both of which usually feel warm.

- The child appears pale (although sometimes the face can appear to be flushed).
- If the child is conscious, she may be confused or have slurred speech. This occurs because tissue metabolism has altered due to the cold.
- The child may be drowsy and limp.
- The child may be shivering (although this is unlikely in a baby as stated earlier).

First Aid and Treatment

Call a doctor and an ambulance (**dial 999**). If the child is unconscious, go through the ABC routine: is the Airway clear?; is the child Breathing?; check the Circulation – is the child's heart beating? If the answer is no to any of these questions then the child will need to be resuscitated (see Chapter 16).

If the child is unconscious but breathing and has a heart beat then place her in the **recovery position** (see page 66) and talk to her, thus providing reassurance. It is *vitally important* that the child is warmed slowly. Rapid re-warming will result in blood vessels to the skin dilating and the child will then lose more heat. If the child is wet, remove the wet clothing, dry her with a towel and then wrap her in a dry blanket. Cover her with several light layers of blankets and try to get some underneath the child to prevent heat loss to the ground. A baby or small child may be warmed slowly by snuggling her inside your own clothing. Stay with the child during her transfer to hospital.

Raised temperature

A raised temperature can also be referred to as fever, pyrexia or hyperthermia.

A raised temperature is an indication of infection. The body responds to infection by raising the temperature as a defence mechanism.

How to Recognise the Child with a Raised Temperature

- She will be irritable, miserable and may be cross – she may be more clingy than usual.
- She will feel hot and appear flushed.

- She may be thirsty and appear to be dry around the lips.
- Despite feeling hot she may shiver – this is because in an attempt to lose heat the body sweats and the sweat cools the skin, which may make the child feel cold and therefore shiver.

It is important to reduce the temperature in a child for two reasons, it will make her feel much better and it will reduce the risk of febrile convulsion (see page 65).

METHODS OF REDUCING THE TEMPERATURE

Cool the child

Heat is lost through the skin by evaporation and radiation. It is therefore important to keep some of the skin in contact with the air. If the child is in bed, remove some of the bedclothes. If she is dressed, remove some of the outer clothes, remembering to ask the child's permission and giving her an explanation. An infant may be left in a vest and nappy and a child in her underclothes, or if she does not feel this is acceptable, then lightweight cotton clothing. Cotton is the ideal choice of material as it is cool to wear.

Keep the room cool, open the window and allow air to circulate; in winter turn the heating down.

Careful observation of the child will allow the carer to be aware if the child is becoming too cool, in which case some clothes may need to be replaced.

Fluids

The child will feel hot and thirsty. Plenty of cool drinks should be offered as these will help to reduce the temperature. A breast-fed baby should be put to the breast more often. A bottle-fed baby should be offered cool drinks, such as cooled boiled water (flavoured if necessary). Milk should be offered in the usual way. A toddler should be offered drinks at least hourly and encouraged to take them. This may mean lots of cajoling but it is very important. Ice lollies are usually very popular with children and they provide an excellent source of cool fluid.

Medicines

Paracetamol preparations are very efficient at reducing the temperature in a child. They can be bought at a chemist and should be stored in a locked medicine cupboard.

Early years workers are advised that medicines should not be given unless the written permission of the parent or next-of-kin is obtained (see Chapter 8).

Elixirs or syrups are recommended for young children (and can be given to older children who have difficulty in swallowing tablets). It is important to follow the instructions given on the bottle.

Babies under the age of three months should not be given paracetamol preparations unless advised by a doctor or health visitor.

Aspirin – or any medicine containing aspirin – should not be given to children under the age of twelve years.

Tepid sponging

This is a method used to reduce a temperature over 38.5°C. This is particularly important if the child is very irritable or if there is a history of febrile convulsions. Tepid sponging should be carried out in a draught-free room, using the following procedure:

- Tell the child in language she understands what you are going to do and speak to her kindly – she is not feeling very well at this stage and needs reassurance. Tell her that what you are going to do will make her feel more comfortable.
- The child can remain in her underclothes. Pour water into a bowl. The temperature of the water should be a few degrees lower than that of the child. Use several sponges. Place a damp sponge in each armpit. Using another sponge, squeezed in such a way that it retains much of the moisture, wipe it gently over the child's skin leaving a layer of moisture. This moisture will evaporate, thus cooling the child.
- Repeat this procedure, changing the sponges every few minutes so that as they get warm they are replaced with cooler ones.
- Sometimes, an older child may prefer to have a cool bath, in which case run a shallow bath with the water a few degrees lower than the child's temperature. Gently help the child into the water and *stay with her.* This has the effect of cooling the child and making her feel more comfortable. Take her out after a few minutes and gently pat the skin dry.

It is important to cool the child slowly as she might start to shiver which will increase the temperature.

Febrile convulsions

A febrile convulsion is a fit which occurs in response to a rise in temperature. Generally this type of response occurs only in children under the age of five years, and it is seen in approximately one in twenty children.

If the child has had one febrile convulsion, there is an increased risk that she will have another one and it is therefore important to take care to cool the child when she develops another raised temperature.

A child having a febrile convulsion will become rigid, and then the body will start to jerk and twitch and the eyes may roll backwards. This will only last a short time (one or two minutes). Some children will be incontinent of urine or faeces during a convulsion. When the convulsion is over the child will either go straight to sleep, or wake and then go to sleep.

FIRST AID AND TREATMENT

You cannot alter the course of the fit. Therefore:

- **stay with the child and prevent her from injuring herself**
- **loosen any tight clothing around the neck, tummy or chest**
- **talk to the child soothingly, giving her reassurance**
- **place the child in the recovery position (see Figure 23) once the convulsion is over and call the doctor**

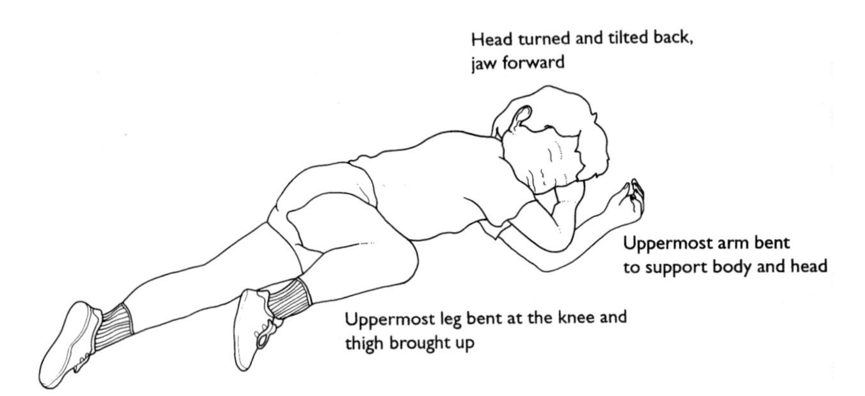

Figure 23 The recovery position

- **start to cool the child by removing some of her clothing and opening a window**
- **if there is anything in the mouth it must be removed, as there is a risk of choking.**

Although it is frightening to watch, the fit will only last a couple of minutes. However, it is important that the carer stays calm.

ACTIVITY

You are a member of a sub-committee in the day nursery and you and the other members of the committee have been asked to review the record keeping.

You have recently cared for a child in the nursery who had a febrile convulsion. The staff were unaware that she was prone to having convulsions in response to a raised temperature. You are keen to ensure that this does not happen again and therefore you wish to amend the registration details accordingly.

What information do you think needs to be incorporated into the initial registration, and how should records be updated to ensure that the early years workers had the required information?

Discuss this in small groups.

Needs of carers when the child is unwell

The nature of the illness will have an effect on the reaction of the carers. A parent of a child with a chronic (long-term) condition may have to make adaptations in many aspects of daily life in order to meet the needs of the child. A parent of a child with an acute illness (one that has a sudden onset) may have to make short-term adaptations in order to care for the child.

The demands of caring for a sick child may be categorised into physical, psychological and possibly financial demands.

Physical demands

Caring for an ill child is physically demanding. Depending on the nature of the illness the child may need to be carried or lifted from one place to another and it is important that carers are aware of good lifting techniques. A child cared for near the main room of the house allows the carer to get on with essential work at the same time as caring for the child. Adaptations to the house may be necessary if the child has a long-term illness, such as muscular dystrophy.

The parent may need to learn new skills from the supporting professionals, such as giving injections to a child newly diagnosed with diabetes. A working parent will need to arrange to take time off work which may cause stress and anxiety.

Psychological demands

It is important to appreciate that a sick child often causes carers a great deal of anxiety. Doctors and other professionals understand this and are happy to discuss such worries.

Anxiety may be caused as a result of past experiences, for instance, if another child in the family had an illness with similar characteristics and was later hospitalised the carer may worry that this scenario will be repeated. Sometimes there is a great deal of anxiety, for example, when there has been an outbreak of an illness such as meningitis in the locality.

Financial demands

Parents who take time off work may in some circumstances risk losing their jobs. Sometimes a parent will have to give up work to care for the child and therefore there will be a drop in income. This may have far-reaching effects on the family. It may mean that the family needs support and guidance in making claims for income support.

Grants are sometimes available for home adaptations that encourage a child to be more independent and advice should be sought.

The early years worker

Physical and psychological demands are also made on the early years worker. It should be remembered that early years workers often build up close relationships with the child, particularly if they work as a nanny. Parents should take time to support the early years worker and discuss some of the implications with her.

ACTIVITY

Go to your local post office and collect any leaflets giving information about financial support for parents of children.

Read the leaflets and make a table that you could use in your profession if a parent came to you for advice about where to go for further information.

Conclusion

Caring for ill children is an extremely demanding role and one that carries anxiety. Whilst meeting the needs of the child it is important that the carer seek help and advice from the professionals should the demands become too much.

8

Medication

Medicines fall into two categories; those that can only be prescribed by a doctor and those that can be bought without a prescription.

Employers have a responsibility under the Health and Safety Act (1974) to ensure that there is a health and safety policy in the workplace. This written policy should include procedures for giving and storing medication and should spell out the importance of careful record keeping and gaining written permission from a parent.

ACTIVITY

Find out the policy on administration of medicines in your workplace and discuss its implications with your supervisor.

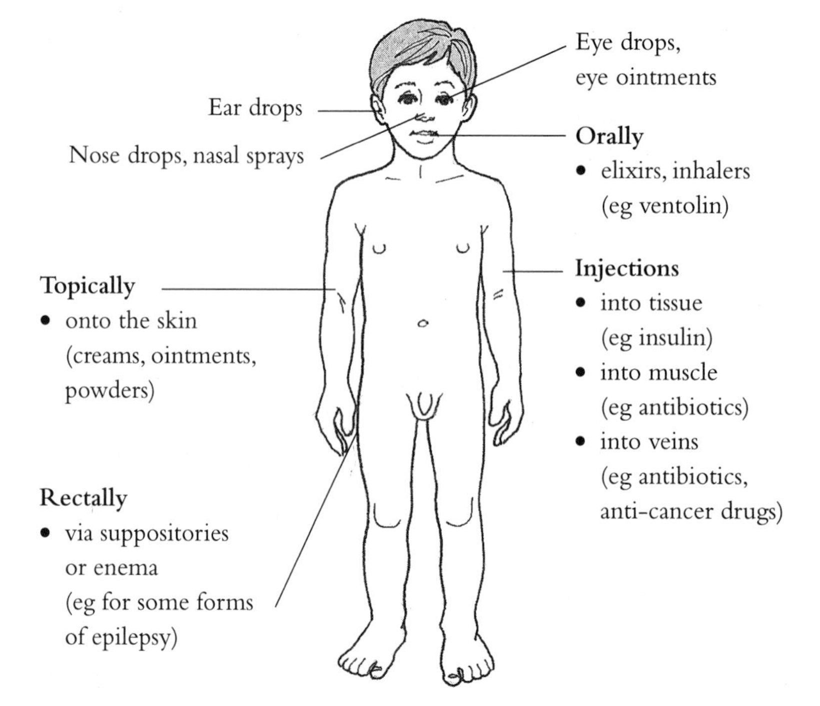

Figure 24 Administration of medicine

Some professionals such as teachers have conditions of employment which do not include the giving or supervising of medication. However, all staff who agree to give medication should have training and guidance. It is important that if medication is given, the person who administers it is aware of common side effects of that medication and knows what action to take if necessary.

In schools the school nurse may provide the training, in day nurseries it may be wise to approach a health visitor for guidance. In some establishments specialised medication such as rectal valium needs to be administered periodically and training is required for this.

ACTIVITY

Find out the desired effects and the side effects of the commonly used medications *paracetamol* and *amoxycillin*. Make a list that you can keep for easy reference.

Record keeping

If a parent asks the early years worker to give their child medication and this is agreed then the parent has a responsibility to provide the following information about the medication:

- Name of the medication.
- Dose (an appropriate measure should be provided).
- The route for administration, for example, via an inhaler or orally.
- Time it was last administered.
- Time for next administration.
- A description of the common side effects.

In the case of medicines that are given 'as necessary', the parent should explain the signs and symptoms that the child might show in order for the medication to be required. For example, with paracetamol elixir – which may be given to lower the temperature – the parent might give permission for administration if the temperature goes above 37.5°C. However, it must be pointed out that the recommended dose should not be given more frequently than six hourly.

The time and the dose of medication given should be recorded by the early years worker and a copy should be given to the parent.

Storage of medicines

Medicines can be harmful if taken by someone for whom they are not prescribed or required. The employer or employing authority has a duty under the Control of Substances Hazardous to Health Regulations (1994) (COSHH) to ensure that the risks to others are controlled. It is therefore important to store medicines in a locked cupboard, with two exceptions:

- asthma inhalers which need to be accessible to the child but not accessible to other children; and
- medications which should be stored in a fridge, such as insulin. The fridge should be kept locked.

Medication should be supplied in a container labelled with the name of the child, the name of the medication, the dose to be given and the frequency of administration.

Oral medication

Medicines are usually dispensed in liquid form (elixirs) for children under the age of twelve. The liquid is flavoured to make it as palatable as possible. Shake the bottle before the dose is measured. The dose will be clearly stated on the label. Non-prescribed (over-the-counter) medicines print age-related instructions for doses and these must be followed. *It is vitally important that the doses are given as directed, both in terms of amount and frequency.*

Medicines should be poured with the label uppermost so that the instructions are not obliterated if a drop of medicine runs down the side of the bottle.

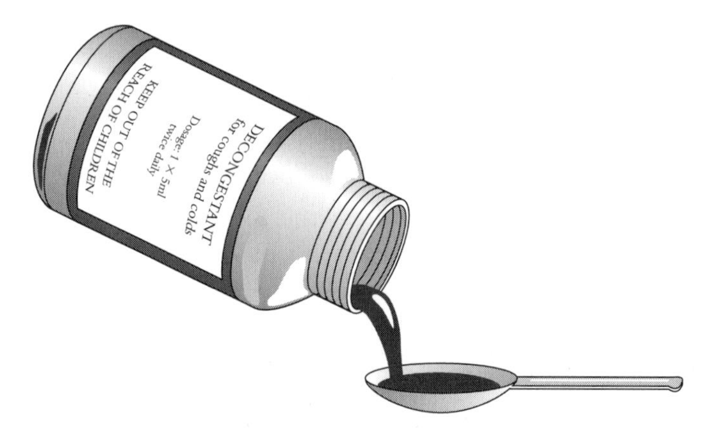

Figure 25 Elixirs should be poured from the bottle with the label uppermost

When the dose to be given is 2.5 ml or 5 ml (or multiples of 5 ml) a spoon is supplied with the medicine. This spoon is shaped in such a way that 2.5 ml and 5 ml measures are both on the same spoon. When the dose is less than 5 ml and not 2.5 ml a liquid medicine measure is supplied.

How to use a liquid medicine measure

1. The liquid medicine measure is marked in 0.5 ml amounts up to 5 ml.
2. It is supplied with a rubber bottle adapter: fit it into the neck of an opened medicine bottle, once the medicine has been thoroughly shaken.
3. Fit the liquid medicine measure into the bottle adapter.
4. Turn the bottle upside down. Withdraw the plunger until the prescribed dose is in the measure.
5. Transfer the medicine to a spoon and give in the usual way to the child.

After use, the measure and adapter should be carefully washed and left to dry. If the measure has been used for a baby, it is recommended that it is sterilised, with the baby's bottle.

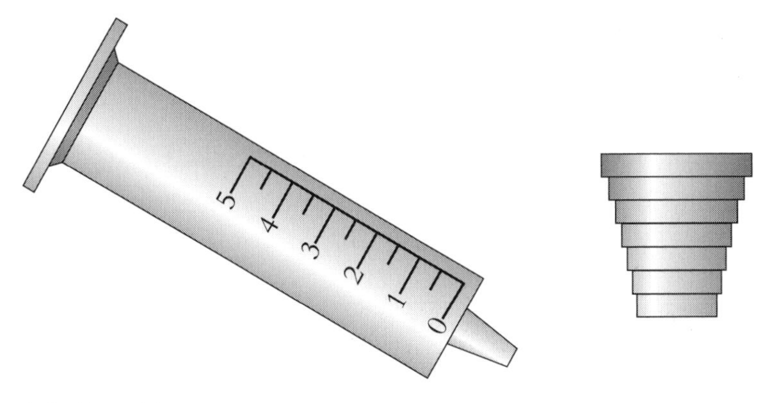

Figure 26 A liquid medicine measure

ACTIVITY

Familiarise yourself with the liquid medicine measure.

Administration of oral medication

Identify the child correctly and match the child with the medicine. This may sound obvious but in some circumstances it may be that several children require medicine at a particular time and great care must be taken to prevent mistakes. Take along another early years worker to act as witness if that is the policy of the establishment. This should not be too intimidating to the child as several activities are undertaken with more than one early years worker.

Prepare the child:

- use language that she understands
- tell her that it is time for her medicine
- be quietly persuasive
- if the child is co-operative ask her to sit down while the dose is measured out
- offer the medication on a spoon and ask her to swallow it
- have a favourite drink ready to follow the medicine
- praise the child for co-operating
- if the child is less co-operative a firm approach may be needed. The early years worker should use all her powers of persuasion to encourage the child to co-operate as this minimises the risk of choking on the medicine. It may be that bribery has a place here – 'if you take this now without making any fuss then you can . . . afterwards' – but always keep your promise
- if the child cannot be cajoled then the parent should be informed and asked to deal with the situation. The early years worker should not force the child to take the medicine.

If the child really finds the flavour of the medicine unpalatable, it might be possible for the doctor to prescribe a similar medicine with a different flavour.

Note: Never pour the medicine into a drink, as if the child does not finish the drink you will have no idea how much of the dose has been taken.

Medicines are usually given between one and four times a day, and some medicines must be taken after food. It is important to space the doses out as much as possible during the twenty-four-hour period but it is generally not a good idea to wake the child at night, unless specifically instructed to do so by the doctor, as sleep is very beneficial to an ill child.

Administration of eye drops

- Wash your hands.
- Reassure the child.
- Place a young child on her back; an older child may be happy to co-operate by holding her head back.

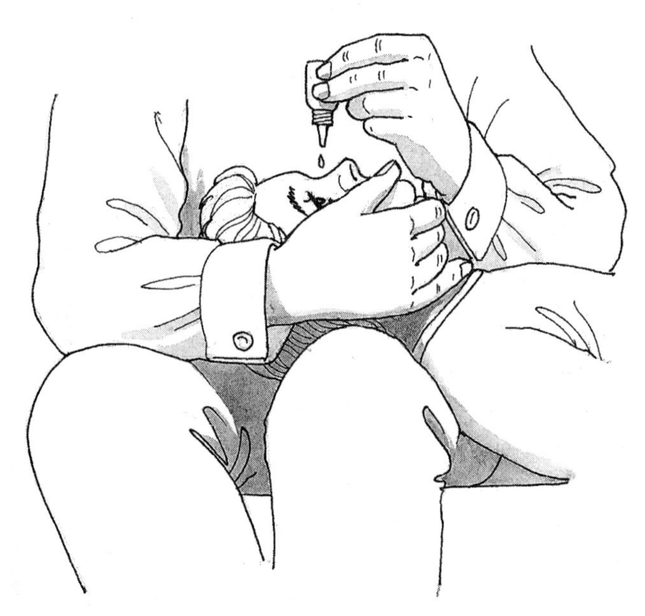

Figure 27 Administration of eye drops (1)

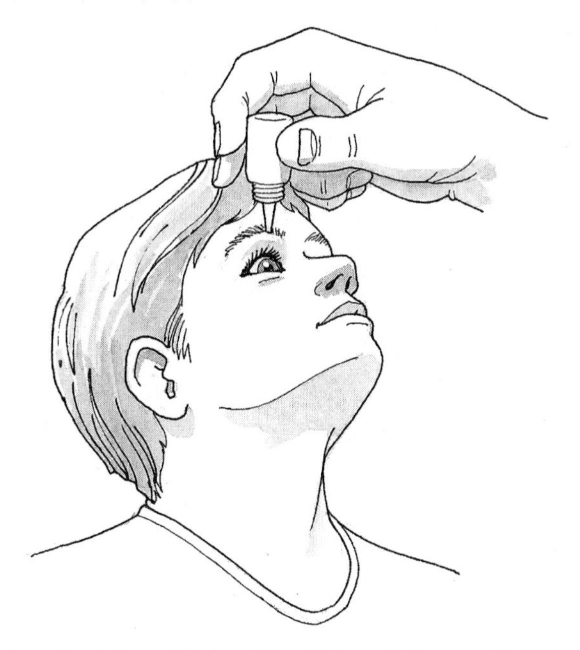

Figure 28 Administration of eye drops (2). An older child can sit down and hold her head back

- Load the dropper and then hold it upside down so that a drop forms at the end of it ready for administration.
- Gently pull down the lower eyelid and place the prescribed number of drops in the space between the eyeball and the lid. It is only possible to administer one drop at a time because the child will blink. Alternatively a drop could be placed in the corner of the eye when it is closed and the child then encouraged to blink.
- Gently mop away any fluid that runs out of the eye.
- Praise the child.
- Wash your hands and replace the eye drops in the correct storage area – often the fridge.

If it is possible to have two people when giving the drops it can be helpful.

Administration of ear drops

- Wash your hands.
- Reassure the child.
- Place the child on her back with the head turned so that the affected ear is uppermost.
- Load the dropper and then hold it upside down so that a drop forms at the end of it ready for administration.

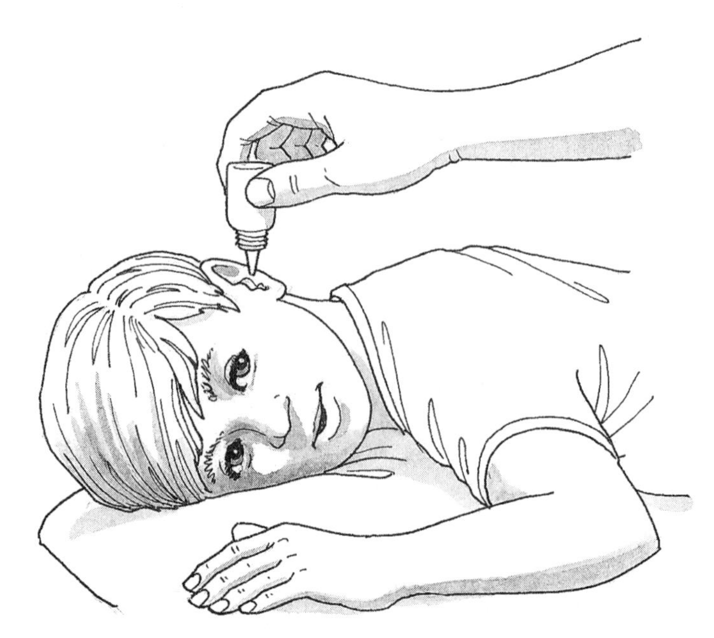

Figure 29 Administration of ear drops

- If the person administering the drop gently rests her hand on the child's head just above the ear and gently pulls the pinna (earlobe) upwards the prescribed number of drops can be given. The child should keep her head still for several minutes after administration.
- Gently mop away any fluid that runs out of the ear.
- Praise the child.
- Wash your hands and replace the ear drops in the correct storage area – often the fridge.

Administration of nose drops

- Wash your hands.
- Reassure the child.
- Place the child across the early years worker's knee with the child's head extended.
- Load the dropper and then hold it upside down so that a drop forms at the end of it ready for administration.

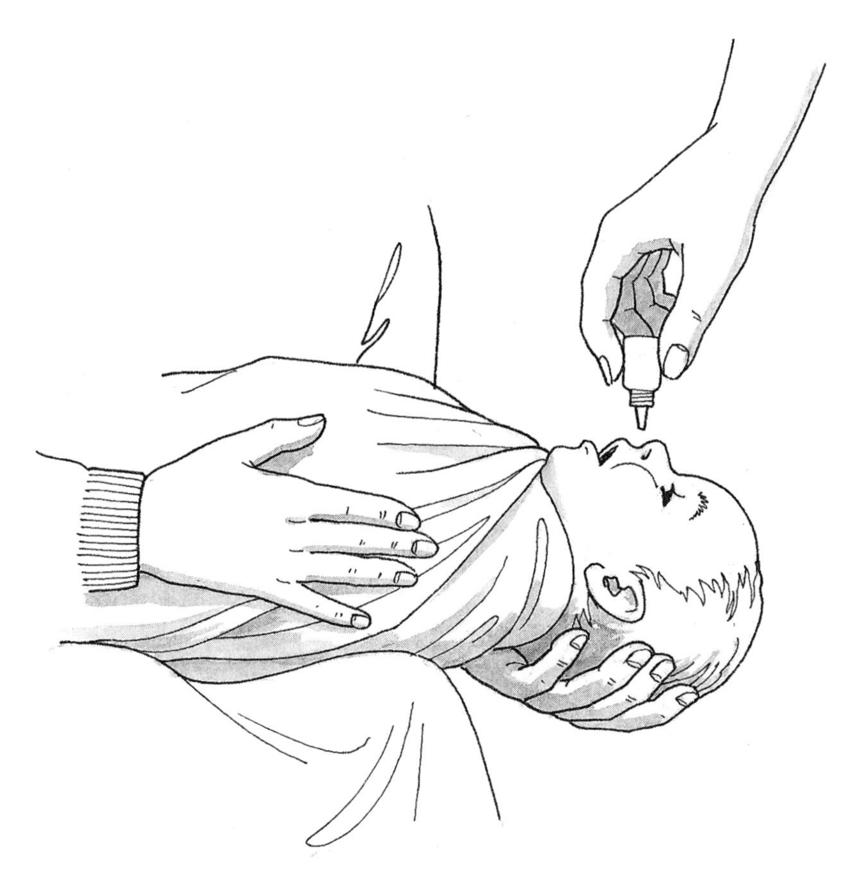

Figure 30 Administration of nose drops

- Place the dropper near to the nostril and administer the prescribed number of drops (one at a time if more than one).
- Encourage the child to stay in the position for about one minute.
- Gently mop away any excess fluid.
- Wash your hands and replace the nose drops in the correct storage area.

Administration of topical medicines (creams and ointments)

A cream or ointment may be prescribed for various skin conditions. Instructions must be followed. The early years worker should wear disposable gloves to prevent absorption of the ointment.

Rectal administration

Very few prescribed medicines in Britain are given rectally. However, sometimes if a child has epilepsy and 'one fit runs into another', a rectal administration of the prescribed medication may be needed. In general, rectal medicines are given by a trained nurse or doctor. However, if an early years worker is in charge of a child with epilepsy, it may be necessary for the employer to teach her the technique.

Injections

The early years worker may find herself looking after a child who requires injections. This skill requires specialist training. If this skill is to be part of the workload, the employer will need to arrange this training with a doctor or nurse.

The medicine cabinet

In the day nursery, playgroup, school, etc., there will be a first-aid box. The workplace will have a set policy as to the contents of that box, and the early years worker should make herself familiar with the contents.

In the home, there is often a medicine chest (out of the reach of children), which should be locked and the key kept near at hand (but not actually in the lock). The contents should be checked at regular intervals, and medicines that have passed their use-by date should be discarded.

Conclusion

Administering medication to a child carries a large responsibility. The workplace should have a written policy and the early years worker should familiarise herself with this policy.

Before administering any medication, the early years worker should ensure that she is given full instructions and that she has a sound understanding of the procedure and the effects of the medicine. If she is not completely confident, she should ask for further advice from her supervisor.

The Professionals

The parents

Although not child care professionals in the true sense of the word, it is the parents who provide the majority of care for the child and who usually have the child's best interests at heart. They initiate treatment if the child is unwell by nursing her and, if necessary, by seeking medical advice. They give the child any medicine and carry out the advice given by the doctor. An early years worker employed as a nanny may take over many of these duties.

The Primary Health Care Team

When a child is unwell, the carer may need to ask for advice from a health visitor, general practitioner, or perhaps the nurse in the health centre. These professionals, together with the community midwife and the district nurse, make up the Primary Health Care Team. This team is generally supported by receptionists, and sometimes includes other professionals, such as the school health nurse, the community psychiatric nurse and a social worker. In some areas, there is also a community paediatric nurse attached to the team. These people work together to provide an effective service to clients in the community. The role of the team is not only the care and treatment of people who are unwell, but also health education and health promotion among healthy people. The team may be based on a health-authority-owned health centre or in a privately owned medical centre (the surgery) or they may be based in separate accommodation. However, whatever the accommodation, they meet on a regular basis to discuss the care of their clients. These regular meetings help to ensure that the clients receive a high standard of care.

The roles of members of the Primary Health Care Team

General Practitioner

A general practitioner (GP) has trained as a doctor and then completed another three years' training, including a year as a trainee general practitioner. She is involved with the promotion of health and the treatment of illness.

When a child's birth is registered, the parents receive a card with a National Health number on it. This is taken along to the surgery, and the child can then be registered with the GP of the parents' choice.

In some rural areas, the GP may dispense medicines from the surgery, but in less rural areas, prescriptions need to be taken to the local chemist in order to be dispensed.

Health Visitor

The health visitor is a qualified nurse who has completed a course in health visiting. She is involved in the promotion of health and prevention of ill health.

Within the field of child care, she is particularly involved in antenatal care, postnatal care and the care of the young child. She, together with the community midwife, often run a parentcraft class in the health centre. The health visitor is involved in visiting the newborn and will subsequently see them in the child health clinics. She will be available to offer help and advice on all sorts of matters concerning child care. In particular, she may discuss feeding problems, sleep problems, the crying baby and immunisation.

Practice Nurse

The practice nurse is a Registered General Nurse employed by a group of general practitioners (or a single-handed GP) and is responsible for seeing and treating some of the minor conditions. She may also be responsible for giving advice in clinics, such as the asthma clinic. The nurse may give routine immunisations to children after they have been seen by the doctor.

Community Midwife

The community midwife works with the doctor to provide antenatal care for pregnant mothers and may be involved in delivering babies in a general practice unit, within the district general hospital or possibly at home. The midwife will be involved in postnatal care, usually until the tenth day after delivery, although in some circumstances, this may be extended until twenty-eight days after delivery. The midwife usually works with the health visitor to provide parentcraft classes in the community.

Social Worker

The social worker may have qualified in one of a number of ways, but will have gained the Diploma in Social Work. She is employed by the social services department and may be based in a central office with other social workers or in a health centre. Social workers may be appointed to work as day care advisors or may be involved in child protection and various aspects of family support. The social worker takes referrals from many sources, for example the GP, the health visitor, the school nurse, and also from clients who feel that they need help and guidance. Social workers are also based in hospitals.

Community Paediatric Nurse

A community paediatric nurse is employed in some districts. Nowadays, children who are unwell are discharged earlier from hospital than in the past. This is partly because it is recognised that children find it less stressful to be cared for at home; once trained in the day-to-day management of their child, parents find it easier to care for the family when they are all under one roof; it also releases a hospital bed for another child. The community paediatric nurse works with the family to enable individual care to be given in the child's own home. She will work with other members of the Primary Health Care Team in order to organise the care needed. Children who benefit from this type of care include those who have been in hospital for surgery, appendicitis for example, diabetics and sometimes children for whom strict bedrest has been advised. The specialist knowledge of the community paediatric nurse will be required for day-to-day management of the patient, such as a diabetic child who has developed an infection.

School Nurse

The school nurse, employed by the Health Authority, is a Registered General Nurse who may also have a School Nursing Certificate. In many areas, the school health nurse will divide her time between several schools and will be responsible for assisting with school medicals, health promotion, health education and care of children with special needs. Her responsibilities also include advising the school about managing relevant medical problems and ensuring that the school is aware of current policies on the care of certain conditions. She may be involved in helping the doctor with medical examinations. Some schools (usually special schools) have a school health nurse on the premises at all times.

The school nurse employed by the Education Authority is not necessarily a qualified nurse. Generally, she has a First Aid Certificate. Her role is to deal with day-to-day problems, such as children falling over and grazing their knees or feeling unwell. The Education Authority school nurse will request medical help if necessary and will liaise with the school nurse (employed by the Health Authority).

THE DENTIST

Training for dentistry takes five years. The dentist's role includes the prevention, diagnosis and management of diseases of the teeth, gums and sockets.

THE ORTHODONTIST

The orthodontist specialises in the correction of tooth irregularities and in the alignment of the lower and upper jaws. Children are referred to the orthodontist by the dentist.

The Secondary Health Care Team

In a hospital, there is a wide variety of professionals.

Often, if a child is admitted to a ward, there is a 'Rogue's Gallery' (named photographs of all the staff working on the ward) on the wall as the child enters the ward. These are often necessary, as increasingly professionals are discarding uniforms in an attempt to be less intimidating to the child.

The roles of members of the Secondary Health Care Team

NURSES

There are usually many different nurses on the ward; some are qualified; some are in training to be Registered Sick Children's Nurses, some may be training to be Registered General Nurses and some may be Auxiliary Nurses. It is recommended that eighty per cent of nurses working on a paediatric ward should be Registered Sick Children's Nurses.

At any one time, a specific nurse (the 'named nurse') will be assigned to a child and this nurse will be responsible for the care of the child during her time on duty. Generally, she will have several children in her care and will usually work with the parents or carers to plan and implement the child's care during her span of duty. In some hospitals, the same nurse will be allocated to the child for several days at a time to allow continuity of care. This does have the effect of reducing the number of people to whom the child has to relate. However, in a twenty-four-hour period, the child will need to get to know at least two nurses. Some hospitals operate a twelve-hour shift system and some an eight-hour shift system.

DOCTORS

During a stay in hospital, the child may meet many different grades of doctors. The senior house officer (SHO) is the doctor that the child will see most often. She will have completed five years in medical school and will also have worked as a house officer for a year.

The registrar is senior to the SHO, having worked as an SHO for several years. She either has an additional qualification in paediatrics or is working towards one.

The senior registrar (SR) is, as the name implies, more senior than the registrar and is gaining further experience whilst waiting for final promotion to the position of consultant. The SR may be involved in research as well as working on the wards.

The consultant specialising in sick children is called a paediatrician. She has ultimate responsibility for the patients. The paediatric consultant will usually work in the hospital, but may do home visits if requested by the general practitioner.

OTHER PROFESSIONALS

There may be occasions when the child is referred to other professionals for specialist advice. These may include:

The surgeon

This is a doctor who performs operations, for example if a child has appendicitis.

The radiologist

The child may need some tests before a diagnosis can be made. The radiographer (see below) is the technician who takes X-rays, and the radiologist is the doctor who interprets them. Radiologists also use radiotherapy in the treatment of some conditions, including cancer.

The radiographer

Radiographers have to complete a three-year course and will probably be seen most often when taking X-rays. However, they are also involved in other specialist tests, such as ultrasound tests, which are becoming increasingly common.

The anaesthetist

If a child requires surgery, she may need an anaesthetic, and this will be administered by the anaesthetist.

The physiotherapist

The physiotherapist also has to complete a three-year course and may be involved in treatment in a number of ways. She has experience in treating people using exercise, manipulation, heat, massage or electrical stimulation (such as ultrasound treatment). The physiotherapist is also involved in the care of people with respiratory conditions, such as cystic fibrosis, asthma and bronchitis.

The play specialist

The play specialist is usually a qualified nursery nurse who has had a substantial amount of experience of working with children and may also have completed a specialist one-year hospital play course. Her role is to encourage children in hospital to play, thus helping them to come to terms with hospitalisation and also to accept their condition. Many hospitals now employ a play specialist for each children's ward, and they are a very important member of the team.

The play therapist

Some hospitals employ a play therapist. She will have completed a further period of training and usually works with children who have experienced particularly traumatic situations.

The occupational therapist

An occupational therapist will have had three years' training. She works mainly with children who have suffered a severe injury or who have a disability and helps them to become as independent as possible. Sometimes, occupational therapists may also be asked to work with children who are considered to be clumsy. Sometimes her work will involve the use of special equipment, and she will give advice on any alterations which may be needed to the patient's home. The occupational therapist will usually be based in the hospital but will visit the home as and when necessary.

The audiologist

An audiologist is a health professional who specialises in the diagnosis and measurement of hearing problems.

The speech therapist

A speech therapist has to complete three years' training. She is involved in how the child communicates, which includes receiving communication as well as self-expression. The speech therapist works in the hospital and in the community.

The dietician

These professionals give advice on the importance of a healthy diet. However, their involvement with the care of children lies in the specific advice necessary for children with, for example, diabetes, food intolerance or food allergies. Dieticians usually work both in the hospital and in the community. Training takes three years.

The teacher

Many hospitals have schoolrooms and employ trained teachers. It is particularly important for children who are going to be in hospital for a long time not to miss out on their education.

Non-hospital-based professionals

Other non-hospital-based professionals involved with the care of sick children include the following.

Child and family psychiatric service

This service is community based and is run by a team of professionals headed by a psychiatrist and including a social worker and community psychiatric nurses. Children can be referred to this clinic by a GP or a health visitor, or the family can refer themselves.

A community psychiatric nurse is involved in the assessment and treatment of children (and their families) with mental health problems.

The community clinic

In some areas GPs do not carry out their own child health surveillance. When this is the case, a clinical medical officer will see the children in a community-based clinic. The clinical medical officer is a qualified doctor who has had extra training in paediatrics. Clinical medical officers may also be seen in specialist clinics.

Schools

Teachers will usually have trained for three or four years. Obviously the prime responsibility is to educate the children in their care; however, it may well be the teacher who notices the initial signs and symptoms of illness and alerts the parents to the situation.

The educational psychologist

The educational psychologist will have a psychology degree and a teaching qualification and will have undergone further training. A child may be referred to her for assessment by the school.

Non-statutory help

When a child is unwell the parent will often ask members of the extended family or friends to assist with some daily activities, such as collecting their children from school. Many parents who have been involved in networking with others in the area find that this sort of support is invaluable during times when a child is unwell.

However, there are times when the parent needs support from people who have a deeper understanding of the problems involved, for instance, if the child has a rare condition there may be limited knowledge available, particularly in practical terms. This is where support may be offered from voluntary organisations and self-help groups. Many of these organisations are national and some have local branches. A list of these groups is available from the local library, social services and the Citizens Advice Bureau.

A list of some of these organisations can be found in Appendix 1.

ACTIVITY

You cannot predict when or if a child will be unwell. However, it is accepted that if the child is prepared in some way, they tend to come to terms with the situation more easily.

You are working in a playgroup and have decided to make the theme for the next few weeks 'going to the doctor'.

1 Develop this theme with one or two peers. You could perhaps draw a spider diagram of your ideas.
2 You might like to make a Rogue's Gallery of the people working in the surgeries that the children go to when they are unwell.

3 Invite one or two of the professionals to the playgroup to talk about their role. They might like to take the opportunity to offer some health education to the children.
4 Go to the local library and borrow some books that are relevant to your topic. The children's librarian is often very helpful when groups are doing topic work.
5 Back up the topic with plenty of relevant toys, such as the Fisher Price doctor's set and Playmobil hospital. If your group does not have enough money to buy the toys, find out whether you can get access to a toy library.
6 Perhaps you could turn the home area into a doctor's surgery.
7 The children could be involved in plenty of creative work during this topic: for example, they could paint pictures of themselves feeling unwell.
8 As most children have had some experience of feeling unwell, they are often happy to talk about it, and there is scope for lots of language work.
9 Develop any other thoughts you may have for the topic.

Preparation for visits to health professionals

During the early years most children will visit their general practitioner either for a routine appointment at the child surveillance clinic or because of illness. As a result of these visits the child may need to be referred to a specialist, usually at the local hospital. From the age of two, children are invited to visit their dentist twice a year. A large number of children will be seen in the accident and emergency department of their local hospital each year and approximately one million children each year will be admitted to hospital for a period of time.

These visits can be very frightening to a young child. The buildings are unfamiliar and are full of strangers, some of whom may wish to invade their personal space. With careful preparation these visits can be made less traumatic for the young child.

If the visit is planned there will be time to prepare the child. Unfortunately some visits will be unplanned, for instance, following an accident. It is therefore a good idea to prepare children generally through play both at home and in the nursery or playgroup. There are many toys and games on the market which allow children to act out various scenarios. The Fisher Price medical kit provides much of the equipment the child might see used by the GP and the stethoscope in this kit even allows the child to hear their own heart beat. Fuzzy felt hospital and Playmobil hospital may be used in the preparation for hospitalisation. Teddies and dolls make excellent patients for the child to examine, and these can be used by the carer to explain what is going to happen to the child. There is always a place for the carer to take the role of the patient, for instance, if teeth are to be examined by the 'dentist' there is really no substitute.

Books are usually enjoyed by all children and there are lots of children's books written in such a way that they prepare the child for these visits. The children's librarian in the local library is usually willing to help identify books for different occasions.

Preparation for these visits in the playgroup or nursery can take on a more elaborate form, perhaps with the theme of the term being 'keeping healthy'. The home area can be turned into a doctor's or dentist's surgery, the out-patient department of the local hospital or even the accident and emergency department. First-aid kits can be collected, using general household equipment such as scarves to act as bandages. There is scope for language work as many of the children have visited the doctor, dentist, hospital or other clinics and they can share their experiences. Various health care professionals could be invited to talk about their work and ideally bring some of the specialist equipment to show.

A visit to the local health centre may dispel some of the mysteries of the place and staff will often be more than happy to talk to the children and show them around. A visit to the dentist might decrease anxiety, particularly if the children are allowed to see some of the instruments. The dentist could take the opportunity to talk about dental health care with the children.

Parents and carers can play a bit part in preparations if they take the young child along with them when they visit the doctor, dentist or out-patient department, but only in circumstances which will produce a positive effect. A child who sees an adult coping with the situation can derive reassurance.

Many waiting areas have a range of toys and games which can act as a distraction whilst the child waits for her turn to be seen.

When the child does attend the surgery or out-patient department the professionals are usually careful to reassure her and will often talk to her and ask her to explain the problem. It is a good idea for the carer to allow time for the child to answer and to interpret as necessary. In this way a relationship can be built up. It may be necessary for the carer to interpret what the professional has said so that the child adequately understands.

Conclusion

The child may well be overwhelmed by the number of different professionals encountered during the course of an illness. However, it must be stated that only a proportion of ill children are admitted to hospital, and only a proportion of those will meet all the people mentioned.

Remember much can be done to alleviate children's worry and anxiety caused by visiting professionals and the carer should help to provide the opportunities through play and visits.

10

Growth Monitoring and Failure to Thrive

Regular monitoring of growth provides the professionals with a measurement of the child's progress. Weight, head circumference and length (or height) are the most commonly used measurements of growth.

In the first year of life the baby should be over double its birth weight by the age of six months and have tripled it by the end of the first year. The baby is always weighed at birth and will be weighed regularly by the midwife during the first ten days of life. The health visitor will then weigh the baby during her early visits and thereafter the baby will be weighed each time she is brought along to the child surveillance clinic.

Growth charts

All measurements of growth, weight, length and head circumference should be recorded on growth charts. A growth chart is a graph and examples can be found in the Personal Child Health Record books handed to the parents soon after the birth of the baby. These growth charts are commonly referred to as centile charts. The charts were published in 1993 using data from a British population and therefore children from other countries may not conform to the centiles in the same way. For instance, Chinese children tend to be smaller and therefore lighter than British babies.

The growth chart has a number of curves printed across it. The middle curve is the fiftieth centile. If the reader reads off the age of six weeks on the weight chart and then follows the vertical line up until it meets the middle horizontal line – the fiftieth centile – it means that fifty per cent of six-week-old **term** (where 'term' refers to a baby born at 40 weeks after the last menstrual period) babies will be as heavy or heavier and fifty per cent will be that weight or lighter; the fiftieth centile therefore is an average for that age.

Using the same principle, the ninety-eighth centile line at the top of the chart means that two per cent of babies will be as heavy or heavier and

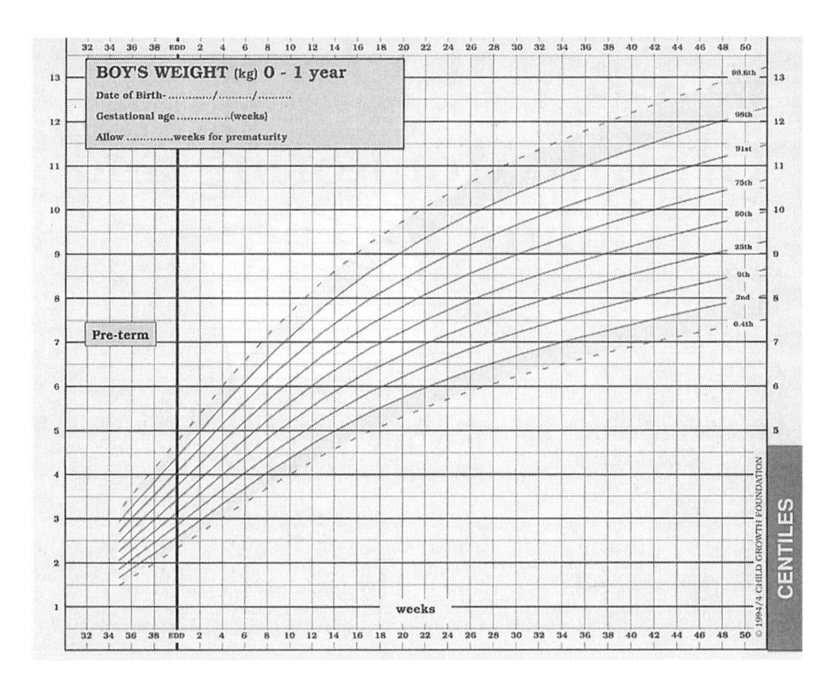

Figure 31 Weight chart

ninety-eight per cent of babies will be that weight or lighter. At the second centile two per cent of babies will be as light or lighter and ninety-eight per cent will be that weight or heavier.

If a baby is born pre-term (prematurely) plotting the measurement must allow for the number of weeks of prematurity. Thus a baby born at thirty-four weeks will have her birth weight recorded at thirty-four weeks. But when that baby is eight weeks old the measurement for weight at that time will be at two weeks after the expected date of delivery time (34 + 8 = 42). Forty weeks is the full term delivery time. This adjustment for prematurity usually continues for the first year of life.

The principles for measuring height and head circumference and plotting the measurements on the charts are the same as described above.

ACTIVITY

Study the growth charts in Figures 31, 32 and 33. Find out your birth weight and mark it on the chart. Parents often keep a record of this information and they may have other measurements that you could plot. Note: If you were born prematurely re-read the information above about plotting measurements.

Reading the charts

It must be remembered that the pattern of growth is the most important aspect when interpreting the growth charts. In general a child's growth curve should run parallel to one of the curves and as long as this is the case the child is usually considered to be growing at a satisfactory rate. Growth is affected by health, and if a baby has a period of ill health she may fall away from her usual growth curve. However, healthy babies will overcome a period of temporary ill health and catch up over the following few weeks.

Crossing a centile band width is a warning to the professionals that there may be a problem. A baby who falls away from the growth curve for weight may be 'failing to thrive' and this will need investigation.

ACTIVITY

Introduce yourself to your health visitor and ask if you could possibly observe some child surveillance clinics. If you are invited then do be aware of the need for strict confidentiality. Observe the weighing, measuring of head circumference and length of babies and recording of them on the centile charts.

HEIGHT

Until the age of one-and-a-half to two the baby is measured supinely (lying down). The first proper measurement of standing height should be taken only when the child is sufficiently co-operative for accurate measurement. Children who are very short or very tall may be at a psychological disadvantage among their peers and the doctor will refer these children to a specialist.

ACTIVITY

'Children who are very short or very tall may be at a psychological disadvantage among their peers.'

Discuss this statement with your colleagues with particular reference to:

- the expectations of adults of a short child with respect to age
- the expectations of adults of a tall child with respect to age
- the 'mothering' of a short child
- the difficulties a tall child might experience when playing with peers.

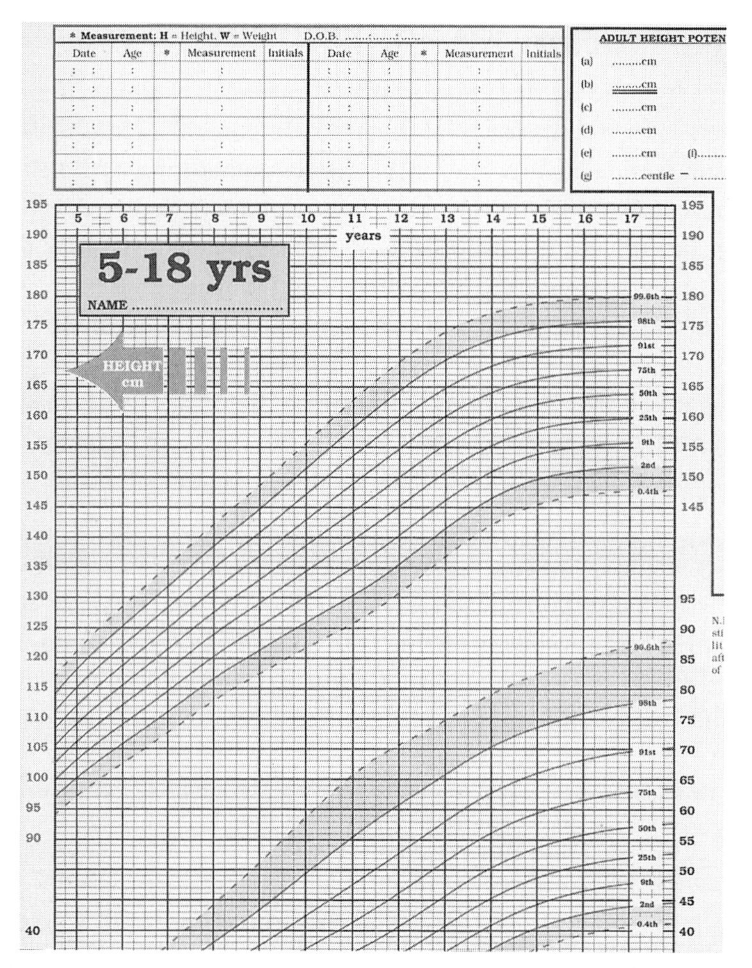

Figure 32 Height chart

HEAD CIRCUMFERENCE

Measurements of head circumference are made regularly and recorded on the appropriate chart. A baby with a rapidly growing head should be referred to a paediatrician as it may be an indication of **hydrocephalus**. A baby with a particularly slow-growing head circumference should also be referred to a paediatrician.

Failure to thrive

'Failure to thrive' is a term used when a child does not conform to the usual pattern of weight gain and growth. A child who is failing to thrive may lose weight or fail to gain weight.

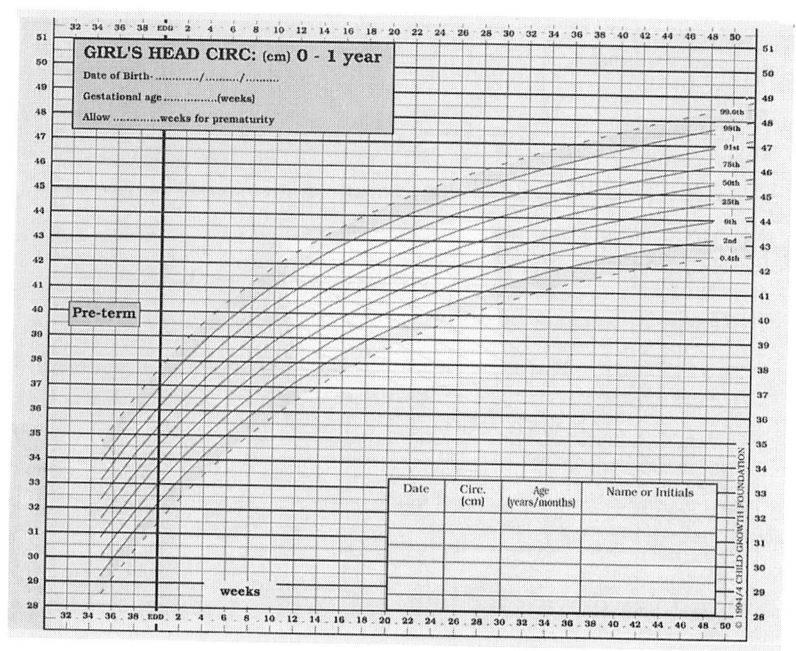

Figure 33 Head circumference chart

Reasons for failure to thrive

If a baby appears to be failing to thrive, the health visitor will usually explore the issues of feeding with the parents in the first instance, as this is the most likely reason for the problem. However, if this proves not to be the case, other avenues are explored. Problems of weight loss or failure to gain weight are easily recognised if the child attends the child surveillance clinic regularly, because a written record of the child's weight is made and plotted on a growth chart. The health visitor will encourage all carers to attend the clinic regularly, particularly if there is any cause for worry. In a recently weaned baby, failure to thrive is most commonly due to intolerance of a newly introduced food. Weight gain – and thus thriving – will occur if the offending food is removed from the diet. This is usually a temporary measure, and the food may be reintroduced at a later stage when it will perhaps be tolerated.

Diagnosis of failure to thrive is made initially by the doctor or health visitor in the clinic. The child may then need investigation, which might require hospitalisation.

A child who is failing to thrive may lose weight or fail to gain weight. This may be due to any of a number of the following:

- poor nutritional intake
- illness and congenital abnormalities not accounted for by poor nutrition
- poverty
- child abuse, including neglect
- hormonal deficiency
- developmental delay.

POOR NUTRITIONAL INTAKE

Causes of poor nutritional intake include:

- problems associated with feeding
- breathing difficulties
- vomiting
- malabsorption of food.

Problems associated with feeding

Usually the health visitor will discuss the possibilities with the parent at length and steps will be taken to rectify obvious misunderstandings, such as making up a bottle feed incorrectly. If, however, the problem is less easily identified, it may take all the skills of the health visitor to try to identify the problem, and if she is not successful, the child will need further investigation. (See Figure 34 for a guide to potential nutritional problems.) The baby may have difficulty with sucking because of breathing difficulties (see below), a cleft palate (which can often be overcome prior to surgery by the use of a specially designed teat or nipple shield) or because of the lack of sucking reflex (some babies born prematurely may not have a very good sucking reflex).

ACTIVITY

You have been asked to demonstrate how to make up a bottle feed to mothers-to-be at a parentcraft class. List the equipment you will need. Which formulas will you take along for demonstration purposes? Give your reasons.

You will need to stress the importance of making the feed up according to the manufacturer's instructions. How do you plan to emphasise the importance of this?

You may have the chance to evaluate your session. Plan a written evaluation form that may be used.

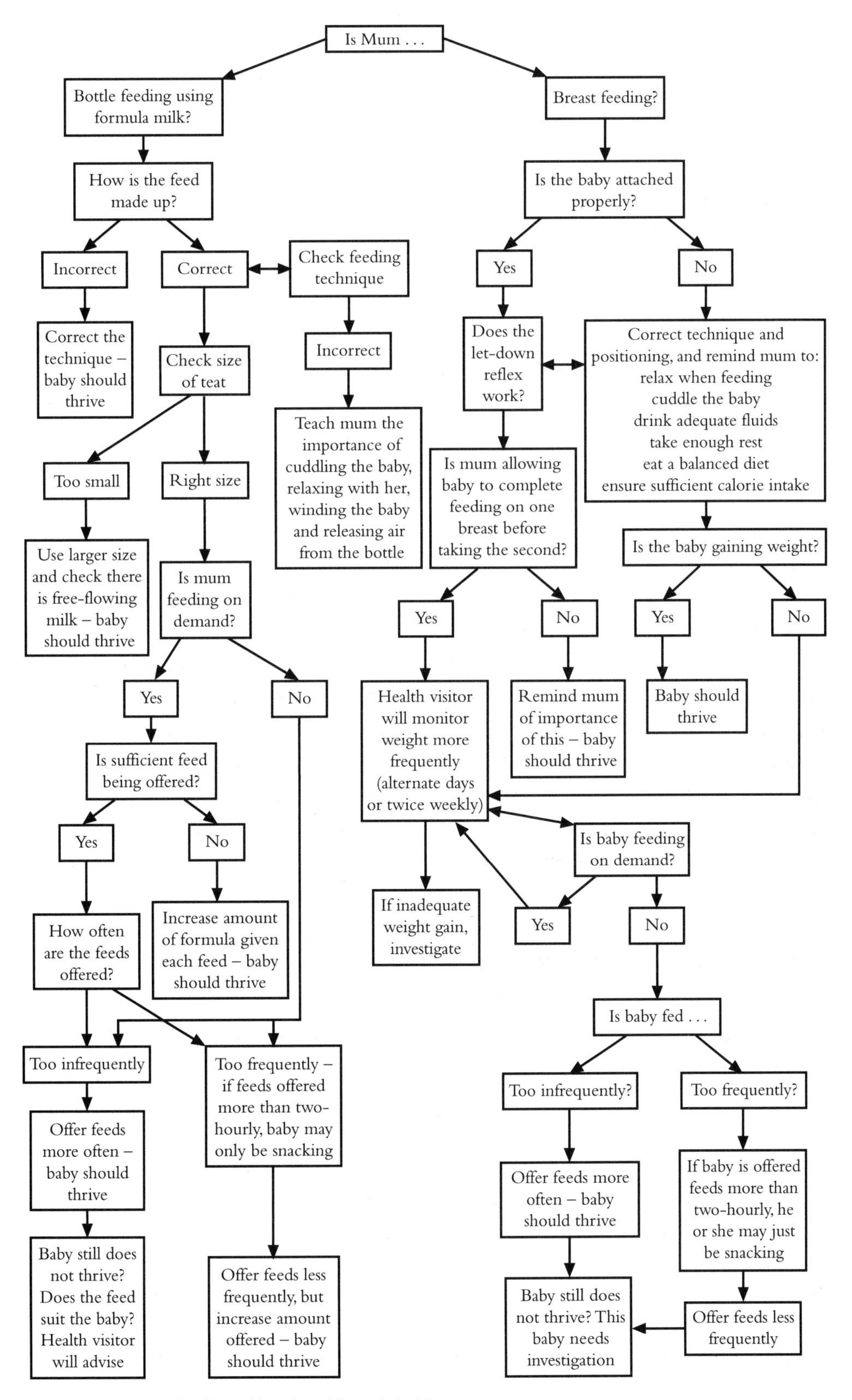

Figure 34 Diagnosis of nutritional problems in babies

Breathing difficulties

Breathing problems may make it difficult for a baby to suck adequately. She needs to be able to breathe through the nostrils while sucking. The common cold can cause temporary blockage, and the general practitioner may, in some circumstances, prescribe nose drops to be used as directed until the blockage has resolved. (This is only a temporary cause for failure to thrive.)

Vomiting

A child who is vomiting frequently over a period of time is unlikely to thrive. Reasons for vomiting include:

Pyloric stenosis This is a congenital abnormality in which the pyloric sphincter (the muscle controlling the point where the duodenum and stomach join) is thickened and narrowed. The undigested milk cannot all pass through, and projectile vomiting results. This condition usually presents itself early in the child's life and can be corrected by surgery.

Hiatus hernia This is due to a weakness in the diaphragm which results in a portion of the stomach being pulled up into the thoracic (chest) cavity. The cardiac sphincter (the muscle controlling the point where the oesophagus and stomach join) is therefore not working effectively, and the stomach contents flow back into the oesophagus (gullet). This condition can usually be corrected by surgery.

Gastroenteritis This is an infection of the gastro-intestinal tract which results in diarrhoea and or vomiting. It is highly infectious.

Whooping cough This is an infectious disease in which the paroxysms of coughing may result in the child vomiting. If this occurs, it is important to offer another feed.

Malabsorption of food

Any child who is not adequately absorbing food will fail to thrive. This condition tends to become apparent after weaning.

Coeliac disease This condition is caused by an intolerance to gluten (a protein found in wheat and some other cereals). Gluten has the effect of flattening the villi (the finger-like projections found in the small intestine), thus impairing absorption of food. The child will fail to thrive and will often be miserable. She may have a distended abdomen and pass frequent, foul-smelling stools. Once the condition has been diagnosed and the gluten has been removed from the diet (which includes exclusion of bread, pastry, etc.) the child will thrive again.

Phenylketonuria (PKU) This is a hereditary condition, usually diagnosed by the Guthrie test (a sample of blood is taken from the child via a heel prick) which is routinely done on the seventh day after birth. In this condition, the child is intolerant to phenylalanine (an amino acid which is a basic unit of protein). Treatment involves the elimination of almost all the phenylalanine from the diet to prevent mental handicap developing. Treatment must commence within the first weeks of life.

Galactosaemia This is a familial disease which is caused by an inability to absorb galactose (a nutrient found in milk). It can lead to mental handicap, cirrhosis of the liver and cataracts. After diagnosis, a dietician will advise the family, as treatment involves giving a diet free of galactose or lactose. This condition may be identified by taking a sample of blood from the umbilical cord or by doing a urine test. These tests will be carried out on all babies where there is a family history of galactosaemia.

Of course, failure to thrive may simply be the result of the child receiving an inadequately balanced diet. If the child thrived prior to being weaned, the health visitor should find out about the diet the child is receiving and may need to discuss with the parents the importance of a balanced diet.

Illness

Children may fail to thrive if suffering from long-term illnesses, including the following.

Cystic fibrosis

This is an inherited disease. Secretions in the body are thicker than usual, with the most commonly affected organs being the lungs and the pancreas. In the lungs, the thick, sticky mucus blocks the air tubes, with the result that the child may suffer from repeated chest infections and have difficulty in breathing at times. The thick secretions in the pancreas result in digestive enzymes being unable to reach the digestive tract, thus impairing the digestion of food. The child therefore fails to thrive. Treatment involves giving pancreatic enzymes by mouth in an enteric (protective) coated form so that they are not attacked by the acidity in the stomach, and teaching the parents to give chest physiotherapy on a daily basis.

Cerebral palsy

This is a condition in which part of the child's brain does not function correctly or has not developed normally. This usually results in muscle control and movement being affected. Some of these children also fail to thrive.

Asthma

This is a disease of the lungs. There is increased sensitivity of the air tubes which causes them to swell and thus become narrowed. There is also an increase in mucus production. Many children who have chronic asthma may have slightly stunted growth.

Urinary tract infections

These are fairly common in young children and may be a cause of failure to thrive. Once a child with a urinary tract infection has been treated she should thrive.

Heart disease

This is seen in approximately eight out of every 1000 births. In infants with large defects, the child may fail to thrive; this is partly due to the fact that they are often breathless because of the less effective heart and tend to suffer from repeated chest infections.

POVERTY

An inadequate income may lead to an inadequate diet, which will inevitably have an effect on the child and her ability to thrive. The health visitor will be a key worker and may invite a social worker to visit the family to help them claim for any benefits to which they may be entitled. (Involvement of the social worker in such cases requires consent from the family concerned.)

Poverty can lead to stress within the family, and stress can and often does have a negative effect on the child. Family stress may lead to a lack of stimulation for the child and subsequent developmental delay. In extreme cases, family stress can lead to non-accidental injury of the child.

CHILD ABUSE AND NEGLECT

The term 'child abuse' may include physical abuse, emotional abuse, neglect or sexual abuse.

Physical abuse

The child may be physically injured, or the injury not prevented, by a parent or carer. This form of abuse may also include giving a child poisonous substances (alcohol, inappropriate drugs, etc.) or attempting to suffocate or drown the child. Children who are physically abused may also be nutritionally and emotionally neglected. Failure to thrive and developmental delay may be the presenting factors in the child clinic.

Emotional abuse

The child is psychologically ill-treated, which, in time, affects her behaviour and development. The parent or carer of an emotionally abused child will continuously fail to show the child affection and love or will shout, bully, reject or threaten the child so that she loses self-confidence and self-esteem. The ill-treatment may lead to failure to thrive.

Neglect

The child may have been persistently or severely deprived of essential needs. There are numerous reasons why parents may neglect their children: for example, if the baby is unwanted, if the parents have not established a good bond with the child or if the mother is suffering from depression or mental illness. The first sign of neglect in these children may be that they fail to thrive.

Sexual abuse

The child is forced to take part in sexual activities which may include intercourse, masturbation, fondling or exposure to pornography. These acts may lead to unhappiness and to failure to thrive.

These causes of failure to thrive can occur at any time in the child's life, but are most commonly seen in the first five years, with the majority of cases being seen in children under the age of one. The child's weight will fall away from the expected centile curve. The child may be disinterested in eating (although she will usually eat readily when in hospital) and may appear to have lost interest in activities previously enjoyed – she may appear to be a rather sad child. Once these children have been identified, they may be put on the child protection register so that they are then regularly checked on.

Children may be abused because parents or carers:

- do not meet the needs of the child
- do not protect the child
- harm the child.

Recognising abuse – the role of the early years worker

Each area in the UK has a child protection committee. Through this committee, procedures have been established.

If an early years worker suspects that a child has been abused, this suspicion must be reported. If the early years worker is working in a junior position, the suspicion may be initially discussed with someone in a more senior position. It will then need to be reported to the social services department, police or NSPCC. The early years worker should write down her observations and include the date and time, a drawing of any injuries and notes and records of what is said. The child is protected by the Children Act (1989).

Note: This section on child abuse is not a comprehensive guide for early years workers, but merely serves as an introduction. The early years worker is advised to attend a course on child abuse. Social services often organise the courses. The local library will be able to obtain books on the subjects. Ensure that you are familiar with the Children Act.

HORMONAL DEFICIENCY

Hormonal deficiency is uncommon in childhood; however, when there is a deficiency, such as with hypothyroidism, there may be an effect on intellectual and physical growth.

Hypothyroidism

Hypothyroidism is caused by an under secretion of the hormone thyroxine which is produced in the thyroid gland. This is usually screened for at the same time the Guthrie test is carried out (seven days after birth). If for some reason this test has not been carried out or if the child has developed hypothyroidism at a later stage, it may become apparent because of slowing in growth.

Growth hormone deficiency

Some children have delayed growth because of a deficiency of growth hormone. Once this has been diagnosed, affected children may have regular injections of growth hormone.

DEVELOPMENTAL DELAY

Developmental delay is often not apparent until later in the child's first year. Of these children, some simply show an unexplained failure to thrive.

Conclusion

'Failure to thrive' is a term used to describe many diagnoses. However, it is a problem which can often be identified by the various health care professionals during the child surveillance at the health clinic, and, once investigated, appropriate treatment can be initiated. Frequently, it is the parents who will bring the child to the doctor because they may have noticed that the child is not gaining weight as she should be. The early years worker may also observe a child who is apparently failing to thrive and would need to discuss this first with the parents (if working as a nanny). However, if she is working with children in another setting, any worries would need to be discussed with the supervisor first.

11

Infection and Immunity

This chapter deals with the causes, spread and prevention of infection and the body's defences against it.

Infection occurs when an organism enters the body and causes a harmful reaction. Microscopic organisms capable of causing infection are called **pathogens** ('germs'). Not all micro-organisms are pathogens, for instance, bacteria living in the gut provide a source of vitamins.

Infections are common in childhood and they take many forms depending on the infective organism and the child's own response to it. They occur when the organism gains entry to the body and is not subsequently destroyed by the body's own defence mechanisms. If the conditions suit the organism it will multiply and the child will become unwell, developing signs and symptoms of infection.

Pathogens

There are a number of pathogens that can cause harm and they may be sub-divided into the following categories:

- bacteria
- viruses
- fungi
- protozoa
- parasites.

Bacteria

These are single-celled micro-organisms and are capable of rapid reproduction in the right conditions. They thrive where it is warm and moist and their growth is inhibited by sunlight and antibiotics. They are found everywhere. The majority are harmless to humans and indeed some are beneficial.

Bacteria are a group of micro-organisms that may be further classified according to their shape which is identified by the use of the microscope. If an infection is suspected a sample of infected material such as urine may be sent to the microbiology laboratory so that the offending micro-organism can be identified along with the antibiotic that is effective against that organism. However, for common infections a broad spectrum antibiotic (one that is effective against a number of micro-organisms) may be prescribed by the doctor.

Bacteria are responsible for a wide range of infections and the reader is directed to Chapter 12 where the cause is identified along with the specific characteristics of that infection.

Viruses

These are extremely small and can only be seen via the use of an electron microscope. They are not cells, simply DNA enclosed in an envelope of fat and protein. They can only reproduce by gaining access into a living cell.

Viruses cause infections ranging from warts to life-threatening conditions such as AIDS (Acquired Immuno-Deficiency Syndrome).

Fungi

These are usually larger than bacteria and may be multi-cellular. Few fungi affect humans, but of those that do, ringworm and athlete's foot are the most common. Some fungi live in harmony with the human body and are found on the skin, in the gut and in the vagina. They are kept in check by other organisms and do not cause ill health under ordinary situations. However, at times they multiply and may cause problems, for instance, fungi living in the vagina are kept in check by the bacteria Döderlein's Bacillus, but these may be killed off when the person is prescribed antibiotics. Under these conditions the fungi multiply and cause itching and discomfort.

Protozoa

Protozoa are single-celled organisms. A few of them can cause ill health in humans, the most common ones being the amoebae which causes diarrhoea (more common in Southern Europe), mosquitoes which cause malaria, and toxoplasmosis.

Animal parasites

A parasite is an organism which lives on or in another living organism for part of its lifecycle, causing harm to that organism. Threadworms, insects (for example lice) and roundworms are examples of parasites.

Entry of infection

Pathogens can enter the body in a number of ways. For example, they may be:

- inhaled, for example the common cold virus
- ingested (eaten), for example food poisoning
- inoculated (introduced via the skin), for example organisms that cause wound infections.

Spread of infection

Infection may be spread directly from one person to another, for example, by kissing or sexual contact, or indirectly through such pathways as air, food, soil and fomites (objects that have been contaminated by an infected person and then used by another, for example, cutlery).

Specific and non-specific defences against infection

The body has two main methods of defence against infection from pathogens:

- The non-specific defences.
- The specific defences mechanism.

The non-specific immune system provides physical and chemical barriers to infective organisms and is summarised in Figure 35.

However, in certain circumstances the infective agents are able to overcome these defences and it is then that the more specific defence mechanism becomes effective.

If infective organisms gain entry to the body an inflammatory response occurs. The infective area becomes hot, red and uncomfortable. This results in many blood cells coming into contact with the pathogens and the white blood cells attempting to destroy them.

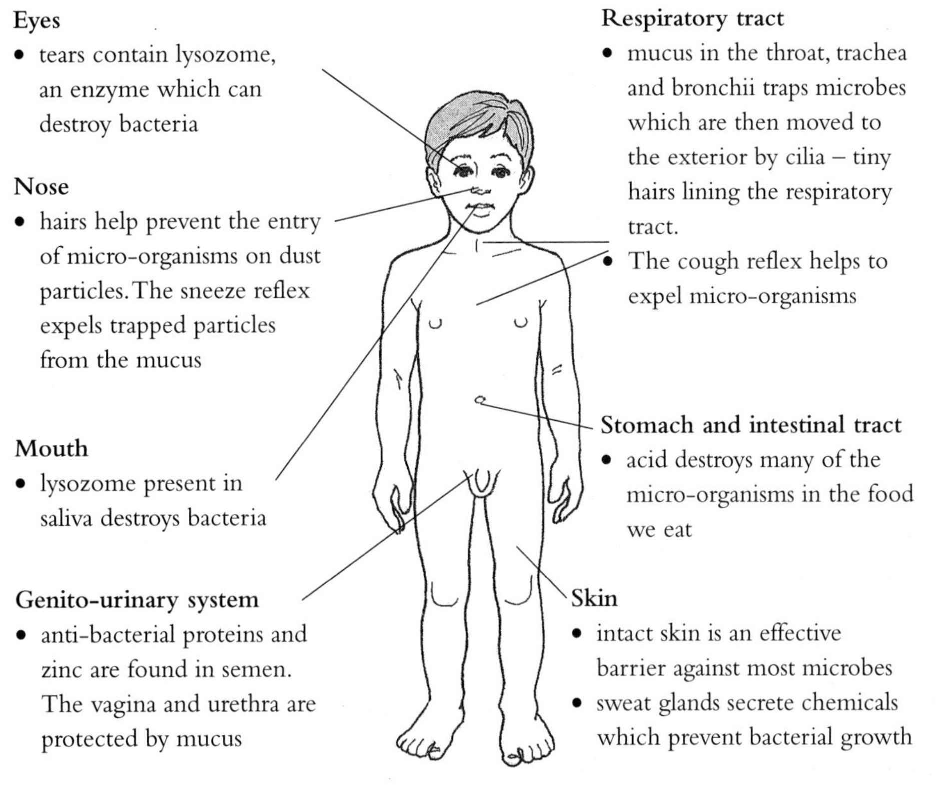

Figure 35 Physical and chemical barriers to infection

The lymphatic system

The lymphatic system has a large part to play in defending the body against infection. It is made up of lymphoid tissue interconnected by lymph vessels. Lymph nodes (see page 47) are widely distributed to cope with the various possible entry points of micro-organisms. Lymphocytes are produced by the lymphatic system and it is these that are the active force. There are two main types of lymphocytes: the B-lymphocyte and the T-lymphocyte.

The B-lymphocytes are involved in the production of **antibodies** which attack the pathogen and so defend the body against illness. The T-lymphocytes multiply in the presence of pathogens and attach themselves to cells that have been invaded by pathogens, and release chemicals to aid their destruction.

When the pathogens have been defeated, the child will regain health. A small number of antibodies remain in circulation, thus providing protection against a further invasion from that particular pathogen.

Immunity

Immunity is the ability of the body to resist infection and may be gained **actively** or **passively**.

ACTIVE IMMUNITY

Natural immunity may be gained by having an infection such as chickenpox, when the virus stimulates the immune system to produce antibodies (see above) and thus the child will overcome the infection. As stated earlier, a small number of the antibodies remain in circulation and will mount a defence if the chickenpox virus attempts to attack a second time. This is a very effective defence and one attack leads to life-long immunity.

Natural immunity may also be gained by having a sub-clinical infection. This is where the infective agent invades the body but does not have enough power to cause a full-blown infection, and the person may be unaware of being infected. However, enough of the infective agent is present to stimulate the production of antibodies and give protection against that particular agent.

Artificial natural immunity is acquired through immunisation. Here the person is given an inactivated (harmless) form of the pathogen, attenuated (weakened) organisms or a modified form of the toxin (the poisonous substance produced by the pathogen) called a **toxoid** which will provoke the immune response and the production of antibodies. Immunisation does not cause disease. Immunity gained through immunisation is generally life-long and is effective against a number of bacterial and viral infections.

- Pertussis (whooping cough) is an example of a vaccine using inactivated organisms.
- Live weakened (attenuated) vaccines include measles, mumps and rubella.
- Tetanus is an example of a vaccine made from toxins which are inactivated.

Immunity is gained after one dose of the vaccine, as in measles. However, in other cases a course of three doses may be necessary in order to build up an antibody response which will be effective against the disease.

PASSIVE IMMUNITY

This type of immunity may be gained naturally or passively. Natural passive immunity may be transferred from mother to baby. During the latter months of pregnancy, antibodies manufactured by the mother cross the placenta thus giving the baby a ready-made protection against the infections the mother has either been immunised against or has had. These antibodies may be further 'topped up' by breast feeding as breast milk also contains antibodies.

This type of immunity gives some protection to the baby in the early months of life but as she has not manufactured the antibodies herself there comes a time when these antibodies are no longer effective. Active natural immunity through having the infection or through immunisation is the only way to secure long-term protection.

Artificial passive immunity may be gained by giving **serum** (the fluid part of the blood that is left when the blood cells have been removed) containing antibodies. These are known as immunoglobulins. This type of immunity is given when the person is not producing enough antibodies or if they are at high risk from an infection, for example a child receiving chemotherapy (see Chapter 17) who is at risk of contracting an infectious disease. Artificial passive immunity gives short-lived immunity but it is effective from the time of immunisation.

Prevention of infection

Babies are more prone to infection than adults because their immune system is in the process of development. There is no set time when this is achieved and for this reason young children as well as babies need to be protected from infection.

All those who have any role in the care of babies and young children must practise a very high standard of personal hygiene and the reader is referred to Chapter 3. It is also essential that a very high standard of hygiene is practised in the home and workplace at all times.

ACTIVITY

You are in charge of a day nursery where student nursery nurses attend for placement. At a recent staff meeting you were asked to take charge of part of the initial induction programme for these students. In particular, you have been asked to ensure that they all understand and practise the high standard of hygiene in the nursery.

Write a list of the areas you feel must be highlighted in the initial meeting and another list of those aspects that can safely wait for a second meeting.

How will you develop this programme?

After the induction programme you will need to ensure that the students maintain these standards. How will you do this without the students feeling that they are being checked up on?

The immunisation programme

The child may be offered immunisations at the child surveillance clinic or during surgery time.

The health professional, the doctor or nurse, will discuss the implications of immunisation with the parents. The aim is to give parents information about the disease and its immunisation so that they can make an informed decision about whether or not their child should have the vaccine. Any specific contra-indications (possible side effects) to the vaccine will be explained.

CONSENT

Once the parents have made a decision it is necessary to obtain written consent to immunisation. The parents will therefore need to sign a consent form, and this will be done at the same time as the general health of the child is assessed. A child will only be given immunisation when she is well.

Figure 36 shows the recommended immunisation schedule for children from birth to eighteen years of age.

CARE OF THE CHILD AFTER IMMUNISATION

Although a few children do have a minor reaction to immunisations, the majority do not. Some children may be whingy and irritable and will need plenty of tender loving care.

Care should be taken not to overheat the child. It is important to ensure that plenty of fluids are given. If an increase in temperature is detected a bath in slightly cooler than usual water may help to bring the temperature back to normal. If this is not effective paediatric paracetamol in the recommended dose may be given. If the carer is unduly worried about the child then advice from the general practitioner should be sought.

The immunisation schedule		
Birth	BCG	given to babies if it is considered likely that they will be in close contact with a case of tuberculosis
two months	Diphtheria Pertussis (whooping cough) Tetanus HIB	given by injection
	Polio	given orally
three months	Diphtheria Pertussis (whooping cough) Tetanus HIB	given by injection
	Polio	given orally
four months	Diphtheria Pertussis (whooping cough) Tetanus HIB	given by injection
	Polio	given orally
twelve to fifteen months	Measles/Mumps/Rubella (MMR)	given by injection
three to five years	Tetanus (booster) Diphtheria	given by injection
	Polio	given orally
ten to fourteen years	BCG	given by injection
thirteen to eighteen years	Tetanus (booster) Diphtheria	given by injection
	Polio	given orally

Figure 36 The immunisation schedule

Sometimes there may be a local swelling around the immunisation site. If it is larger than the size of a 10p it is recommended that advice from the doctor is sought.

ACTIVITY

You are working in a day nursery. The parents of a newborn baby have come to look around the nursery and, finding you to be approachable, they mention that they understand that their baby has to be given immunisations but they are unsure about all the illnesses that the child will be immunised against.

They have asked if you could give a fuller explanation.

Given that this will take some time, you agree to look up information on the diseases and discuss it with them the following day.

Using the information given in Chapter 12 and leaflets you collect from the doctor's surgery, produce a more detailed schedule for them.

Conclusion

Children are particularly susceptible to infections for several reasons: their immune system is not fully developed, they tend to play in close proximity to other children, and they need to be taught and reminded about acceptable standards of hygiene. This chapter has emphasised the carer's role in the promotion of health and the prevention of infection.

12

Childhood Infections – Specific Care and Treatment

This chapter is intended for use as a reference section on childhood infections. The information can be accessed easily as it is grouped according to the area of the body affected. For example, conjunctivitis is found in the section on infections of the eye.

Babies are, to some extent, protected against infection in the first few months of life because they usually have immunity in the form of antibodies, passed from their mothers whilst *in utero* (see page 108). This immunity may be further boosted by the antibodies that are passed through the breast milk if the baby is breast fed. The immunity from these antibodies is relatively short lived, and in time the baby will manufacture her own antibodies in response to infections.

General points

- The incubation period is the time gap between the entry of the micro-organism and the appearance of symptoms. During this period the child could pass the micro-organisms to others.
- Only specific care is included in this section. For general care of the ill child, refer to Chapter 7.
- In many infections the child will have a raised temperature. Refer to page 64 for information on reducing the temperature.
- If you are worried about a child in your care at any time, ask for advice from the health visitor or the general practitioner.
- Children can resume their usual social activities, including school or early years setting, when they are well.
- Immunisation will protect the child against some of these infections.

Common infectious diseases

Chickenpox (viral)

incubation period
13–21 days

time child is infectious
from one day before the rash until scabs have dried

CHARACTERISTICS

A child with chickenpox:

- may be 'off colour' for a few days before the appearance of the rash
- may have a raised temperature and a headache
- will have a rash which starts on the head and behind the ears. This rash eventually covers the whole body. It is characterised by red spots, blisters and dry scabs all being present at one time, once the infection has established itself. The rash is itchy.

SPECIFIC CARE

- Keep the child's nails short so that she cannot tear the skin when scratching.
- Keep the child cool and use calamine lotion dabbed on the skin to reduce itching. Sometimes medication to prevent itching may need to be prescribed.

COMPLICATIONS

Chickenpox usually passes without complications. However, scratching spots may cause them to be infected and result in scarring. Chest infections and rarely encephalitis (inflammation of the brain) may occur.

Mumps (viral)

incubation period
17–21 days

time child is infectious
seven days before swelling and up to nine days after

This is a condition where the virus affects the salivary glands, particularly the parotid glands which are found below the ears.

Characteristics

The child:

- will be 'off colour' for a few days before the more obvious features of mumps become apparent
- may have a raised temperature (which may last up to a week)
- may have a headache
- will develop swelling of one or both parotid glands, causing discomfort
- will have a dry mouth
- may encounter pain when eating and drinking.

Specific Care

- Paracetamol will help to relieve the pain and reduce the temperature.
- The child should be encouraged to have plenty to drink.
- The child may find sloppy foods easier to eat.

Complications

This is usually a mild disease; however, the child may develop mumps meningitis (inflammation of the lining of the brain) or encephalitis. The testes may swell in a boy, and the ovaries may swell in a girl, both causing pain locally.

Rubella (German measles) (viral)

incubation period
14–21 days

time child is infectious
from a few days before the rash until four days later

Characteristics

The child:

- has a rash of small, pink spots (lasting two to three days) and swollen lymph glands at the back of the neck and often elsewhere

- may be a little 'off colour' for a few days before the rash and may have a slight fever.

SPECIFIC CARE

As rubella is usually mild, there is no specific care. However, rubella caught in the first few months of pregnancy can seriously damage an unborn child, causing deafness, blindness, mental retardation and malformations of the heart. Unfortunately, it is infectious for seven days before the rash is apparent, and it is therefore important to inform women of child-bearing age who have been in contact with an infectious child.

Rubella immunisation was introduced for all girls in the UK in 1970. In 1988, it was introduced in the form of MMR (measles, mumps and rubella), and both boys and girls are offered immunisation between the ages of twelve and fifteen months.

COMPLICATIONS

There is a slight risk of encephalitis.

Measles (viral)

incubation period
10–14 days

time child is infectious
from one day before first symptom until four days later

This is an unpleasant and very infectious viral childhood disease.

CHARACTERISTICS

The child:

- is unwell for three or four days before the rash appears
- will have Koplick's spots (small, white spots) on the inside of the cheeks before the skin rash is apparent
- will often have a temperature, a runny nose, red eyes and a cough
- will have a rash, behind the ears and at the back of the neck initially, which then spreads all over the body – the rash is reddish-brown in colour, the spots are flat and joined together and look blotchy
- will often dislike bright light (photophobia).

Specific Care

- Control of the child's temperature is important, as it may rise to 40°C.
- Ensure that the child has plenty of fluids.
- The child will be more comfortable if cared for in a darkened room.

Complications

The child may develop conjunctivitis, otitis media (inflammation of the middle ear), chest infections or encephalitis.

Whooping Cough (Pertussis) (bacterial)

incubation period
7–10 days

time child is infectious
from seven days after exposure until twenty-one days later

Whooping cough is a serious bacterial disease; babies under the age of one are most at risk.

Characteristics

The child:

- will have a cold and cough initially
- may later suffer prolonged bouts of coughing, during which she may have difficulty in breathing
- may go blue at this stage due to lack of oxygen
- will probably make a characteristic whoop at the end of the bout of coughing
- may also vomit at this stage
- will have a cough which may last several weeks.

Specific Care

- A doctor should be called if the child's condition deteriorates or if there is any difficulty in breathing.
- The child should be cared for in a smoke-free atmosphere.
- During a coughing bout, the child should be sat upright.
- The carer should reassure the child during an attack – any panic in the carer may be frightening for the child.

- The child should sleep in the same room as the parents, who will need a lot of patience as the child will be unwell for several weeks.
- The child will need plenty of rest, as the bouts of coughing will disturb her sleep.
- After vomiting, the older child will need a mouth rinse. A baby should be offered another feed.
- Severe cases of whooping cough are admitted to hospital where they are barrier nursed and given specific care.

COMPLICATIONS

The vomiting may lead to loss of weight, malnutrition and dehydration. The child is at risk from many other complications, including pneumonia and bronchitis, which may lead to permanent lung damage, and a hernia because of the severe coughing. Lack of oxygen during a bout of coughing may lead to convulsions. Encephalitis may occur. Babies under the age of six months are particularly prone to complications and may die as a result of whooping cough.

Infections of the nervous system

Meningitis

Meningitis is an inflammation of the meninges (protective coverings of the brain and spinal cord). It is a serious and potentially fatal disease. Meningitis affects children more commonly than adults.

CAUSE

Meningitis can be caused by bacteria (usually meningococcus, pneumococcus or haemophilis influenza type b) and viruses. The viral form of the disease is usually less serious. Note: Haemophilis influenza type b (HIB) has now been almost eliminated by immunisation of infants.

CHARACTERISTICS

The child:

- may become very unwell, very quickly
- will usually have a raised temperature
- will usually have a headache
- may be nauseated or actually vomit
- may dislike bright light (photophobia)
- may have a stiff neck
- may become drowsy

- may have joint pain
- may have a fit
- may have a rash and bruising.

In a baby, it can be more difficult to diagnose, but the following characteristics should be looked for. The baby:

- will usually have a raised temperature
- will often have a high-pitched cry or whimper
- may refuse feeds
- will be very irritable
- may have bulging of the fontanelles (the soft spot on the top of the head)
- may have a convulsion
- may have neck retraction and arching of her back
- may be very drowsy.

Specific Care

- If meningitis is suspected, medical help should be sought without delay.
- If the child is very unwell, she should be taken to the accident and emergency department at the nearest hospital.
- The child's temperature should be reduced to prevent a convulsion (see page 65).
- Darken the child's room.
- Reassure the child and stay calm.

A child with meningitis will be admitted to hospital, where she will be barrier nursed to prevent the spread of infection. The GP may give antibiotics to the child before she is transferred to hospital.

Complications

Meningitis can cause long-term side effects, such as deafness, mental handicap and epilepsy, and in some cases may be fatal.

Prevention

Immunisation against haemophilus influenza type b (HIB) has been available since October 1992. It is offered at the same time as immunisation against tetanus, pertussis and diphtheria. There is currently no vaccination against the other forms of meningitis (bacterial or viral).

Infections of the eye

Conjunctivitis

Inflammation of the conjunctiva (membrane between the eye and the eyelid) caused by bacteria or virus. (Sometimes conjunctivitis may be the result of an allergic reaction.)

CHARACTERISTICS

The child:

- may rub her eyes frequently
- may have a discharge of pus from the corner of the eyes, particularly in the mornings.

The child's:

- eyelids may stick together, particularly after a night's sleep
- eye may be itchy
- eye may weep
- eye will be red.

SPECIFIC CARE

- The child will need reassurance if the eyelids are stuck together, as she may be frightened.
- The carer must wash her hands before and after bathing infected eyes. The eyelids should be bathed gently using warm water and cotton wool. Each eye must be wiped from the bridge of the nose outward, and the cotton wool discarded after each wipe.
- The child should be encouraged to keep the eye closed until the pus has been removed.
- The child will need to be seen by a doctor, who may prescribe antibiotic eye drops if she thinks the cause is bacterial. If the cause is allergic or chemical, anti-inflammatory eye drops may be prescribed.
- If the child is old enough to understand, she should be encouraged not to touch the eyes and, if she does, to wash the hands afterwards.

Remember, conjunctivitis caused by bacteria or viruses is easily spread, so the child should be kept at home until the condition has improved. Face cloths and towels should never be shared because of the risk of infection.

Infections of the ear

Otitis Media

This is an inflammation of the middle ear caused by bacteria or virus.

Young children are more prone to otitis media because of their relatively short Eustachian tube (the tube that connects the throat and the ear). This means that bacteria or viruses in the throat can easily track up into the ear.

CHARACTERISTICS

The child:

- may have recently developed a cold
- may appear unwell
- will usually complain of earache
- will pull at their ears if unable to indicate the pain verbally
- may have a raised temperature
- may vomit
- may have difficulty with hearing
- may have pus discharging from the ear (which occurs if the ear drum perforates).

SPECIFIC CARE

- The child will need to see a doctor, who may prescribe antibiotics and sometimes a decongestant.
- The child will need some paracetamol to relieve the pain and reduce the temperature.

COMPLICATIONS

Some children suffer from recurrent otitis media and may develop glue ear (see below). These children may be referred to an ear, nose and throat (ENT) specialist and may need to have grommets inserted.

Glue Ear

A condition characterised by a build-up of sticky fluid in the middle-ear cavity. This prevents normal vibration of the tympanic membrane and can lead to partial deafness. It occurs most commonly as a complication of otitis media.

CHARACTERISTICS

The child:

- will usually have a history of repeated ear infections
- will probably have intermittent hearing loss, which can be very frustrating for both the child and the carer
- may show a change in behaviour (for example, become very clingy, demanding or disruptive) during these episodes.

The child's:

- speech may be adversely affected (in order to develop a normal speech pattern, children need to hear words clearly – if the sound is frequently muffled, speech may be unclear)
- schoolwork may deteriorate.

SPECIFIC CARE

- The child will need to see a doctor if glue ear or hearing loss is suspected.
- The doctor may refer the child to a specialist, who will arrange further investigations.
- If severe enough, the specialist may wish to insert grommets into the ear drum to aid the drainage of the fluid and ventilation of the inner ear.
- Insertion of grommets is done under a general anaesthetic, and the child will be admitted to hospital.
- Sometimes the adenoids (lymph tissue found in the nose) are removed at the same time, as they may have been contributing to the cause.
- Advice will need to be taken as to whether the child can get the ears wet after the insertion of grommets (opinions vary).
- If the child has speech difficulties resulting from this, she will be referred to a speech therapist.

COMMUNICATING WITH A CHILD WITH A HEARING LOSS

- Gain the child's attention before speaking.
- Speak clearly.
- Keep background noise to a minimum.
- Be aware that the child may not hear you.
- Be understanding. The child may be bewildered by intermittent loss of hearing and need your reassurance.

Infections of the respiratory tract

The Common Cold

A viral infection of the upper respiratory tract. There are many different viruses that can cause the colds, and the child may be infected several times a year.

Characteristics

The child may:

- have a runny nose
- have a sore throat
- have a raised temperature
- sneeze
- cough
- feel generally unwell.

Specific Care

- Make sure that the child has plenty of fluids and rest if unwell.
- Seek medical advice if a baby is having difficulty in feeding or breathing, or you suspect another infection, such as influenza, a chest infection, conjunctivitis or an ear infection.

Croup

This is a condition characterised by a barking cough. It is usually caused by a virus often associated with the common cold. The virus causes the air passages to swell, and breathing is noisy due to the air passing over the swollen respiratory tubes. Attacks occur more frequently at night. The child may have been well when she went to bed.

Characteristics

The child may:

- be hoarse
- have a barking cough and breathe more rapidly than usual
- have difficulty breathing and be fighting for breath
- be distressed and frightened
- wheeze
- drool saliva.

Remember, the combination of rib recession (when the ribs appear to be sucked in), drooling and difficulty in breathing may indicate that the child is very unwell, and urgent medical assistance should be sought.

Specific Care

- Stay calm. If the carer panics, the child will panic, which will make breathing more difficult.
- Ask someone to ring the doctor (and ambulance, if the child is severely unwell). If there is no one else in the house, pick the child up first and hold her while ringing to give reassurance.
- If at any time the child is having serious breathing difficulties, an ambulance must be called. It is advisable to call the doctor as well, as she may arrive before the ambulance.
- Take the child to the bathroom, close the windows and steam the room up by filling the bath with hot water. The warm, moist air, together with the closeness of the carer, often results in a great improvement. *Ensure that the child is kept safely away from the hot water.*
- Stay with the child in this atmosphere for approximately twenty minutes.
- If there is a noticeable improvement, take the child back to her bed or cot. A parent should sleep in the same room and be prepared to repeat the procedure again if necessary. The doctor will have visited or offered advice by this time.

Infections of the chest

These are a group of infections, including bronchitis (inflammation of the bronchi due to infection), bronchiolitis (inflammation of the bronchioles due to infection which affects babies and young children) and pneumonia (inflammation of the lung). Although they affect different areas of the lungs, many of the characteristics are similar. They may be caused by bacteria or viruses.

Characteristics

The child:

- may have a chesty cough, initially dry; later, she might produce phlegm, which children usually swallow
- may have a coughing attack, which may result in vomiting
- often has a raised temperature
- often has a rapid respiratory rate
- will look and feel unwell
- may wheeze

- may be restless and irritable
- may have a dry mouth.

Specific Care

- The child will need to see a doctor.
- If the child is having difficulty breathing, she will need urgent medical attention and an ambulance will need to be called.
- Encourage the child to take plenty of fluids. If breast fed, the baby should be offered the breast more often.
- Prop the child up with pillows if she is in bed. For babies, raise the head of the cot rather than using pillows. Alternatively, breathing will be easier if the child is held in a sitting position, supported and reassured by the carer.
- Allow plenty of rest and sleep. Running around may start a coughing attack.

Tuberculosis (TB)

A condition in which many areas of the body can be attacked by the bacteria. In the UK, seventy-five per cent of new cases affect the respiratory tract. Other areas that may be affected include the kidneys, meninges (membrane enclosing the brain and spinal cord) or bone. The condition is usually found among immigrant families from areas of the world where TB is more common. It is also increasing in the UK particularly in the homeless and in the more vulnerable members of the population.

Characteristics

A child with TB lung may:

- be tired
- lose their appetite
- lose weight
- cough
- have a raised temperature.

Specific Care

The child will be admitted to hospital for initial care. She will have various examinations, and once the diagnosis has been confirmed, antibiotic treatment will be started. Antibiotics will be given long-term (i.e. for up to a year). The child will be reviewed in an out-patient clinic regularly during this time.

Prevention

BCG immunisation is routinely given in some areas of the country at the age of ten to fourteen. Babies born to parents of ethnic background where it is known that the incidence of tuberculosis is high (for example, the Indian subcontinent, parts of Africa and Central and South America) are given a BCG soon after birth.

Infections of the throat

Tonsillitis

Inflammation of the tonsils, which may be caused by a bacteria or virus.

Characteristics

The child:

- will have a sore throat and pain on swallowing
- will have a raised temperature
- will look and feel unwell
- will have enlarged tonsils
- may have unpleasant breath
- may have abdominal pain
- may feel sick or vomit.

Specific Care

- Plenty of rest.
- Fluids should be encouraged – ice lollies are particularly soothing.
- Give pain relief, for example, paediatric paracetamol.
- The child may need to be seen by a doctor, who may prescribe antibiotics. However, the majority of cases are caused by viruses, and the doctor may feel that antibiotics are not appropriate.
- It may be necessary to remove the tonsils (tonsillectomy) if the child suffers repeated attacks of tonsillitis. The child would need to be referred to an ear, nose and throat specialist for advice.

Complications

Very rarely it can lead to nephritis (inflammation of the kidney) or rheumatic fever (an infection of the heart).

Infections of the gastro-intestinal tract

Oral Thrush

This is a fungal infection of the mouth which affects young babies more frequently than older children.

Characteristics

- White patches inside the mouth, particularly on the gums and tongue, which cannot be wiped off.
- The baby may be reluctant to feed.

Specific Care

The baby will need to be seen by a doctor, who will prescribe treatment.

Gastroenteritis

This is a condition where there is inflammation of the stomach and bowel caused by a virus or bacteria.

Characteristics

The child:

- usually has diarrhoea
- may vomit
- often has a raised temperature
- has a loss of appetite
- may have abdominal discomfort.

Specific Care

General

- Gastroenteritis can be serious, and the child should be taken to the doctor if the carer is concerned.
- Children with gastroenteritis should be cared for at home.
- Hygiene must be of a high standard. The infection spreads quickly.
- The child will need reassurance.
- If the child is vomiting, she will need lots of reassurance whilst vomiting and afterwards, when she often feels wretched. The carer will need to protect the area around the child to prevent soiling. A bowl should be provided, and the carer will need to stay with the child. After vomiting, the child should be offered a mouthwash if she is old enough to co-operate. Clothes should be changed if necessary, and the child should be allowed to rest.

- Small amounts of fluid should be frequently offered; the doctor or health visitor may suggest an electrolyte-replacing mixture to prevent dehydration (see below).
- The anal area may become sore – careful washing and the use of a barrier cream will help to prevent this.

For a baby

- Consult the health visitor or doctor. The advice is usually to stop milk feeds. The baby should be offered small amounts of water (preferably mixed with Diarolyte or Rehydrat) at frequent intervals, for example every fifteen to thirty minutes. Diarolyte and Rehydrat can be bought from the chemist without prescription. These are electrolyte replacing mixtures powders that contain glucose and minerals to replace those that are lost through diarrhoea and vomiting. They must be made up as directed.
- Wash the nappy area with care and use a good barrier cream to protect the skin (diarrhoea can chafe the skin, leaving it very sore).
- Nappies should be dealt with carefully, remembering that they contain infective waste. Hands should be washed with soap and water before and after handling them.
- The baby will need more rest. Keep her near you so that you can monitor the situation and be there to help if she vomits.
- The baby may be very irritable, this is understandable, so cuddle her and keep her as comfortable as possible.
- Watch out for signs of dehydration (see below).
- Once the diarrhoea and vomiting has stopped, feeds can be gradually reintroduced. Initially, the feed should be made up at half strength and the baby fed more often than usual, with smaller amounts at each feed; for instance, if the baby usually has 6 oz of feed every four hours, then offer $1\frac{1}{2}$ oz of half-strength feed every hour for a few hours. If this is tolerated, offer 3 oz every two hours and so on, until the half-strength milk is being offered and tolerated at the usual feed times, then gradually reintroduce full-strength milk.
- Breast-fed babies are much less likely to get gastroenteritis. If a breast-fed baby develops gastroenteritis, the parent should discuss the care with the doctor or health visitor.

For older children

- Stop all milk (and milk products) for twenty-four hours.
- Offer Diarolyte or Rehydrat (as above).
- If the child is hungry, offer bland, milk-free foods in small amounts when she has stopped vomiting.

- Encourage the child to have plenty of rest.
- Be particularly kind and patient with the child, as she may feel embarrassed.
- Gradually reintroduce food and milk; discuss with the health visitor if unsure.
- Watch out for signs of dehydration (see below).

Signs of Dehydration

The child will be thirsty. She will pass little or no urine (as a guide, a baby's nappy is usually wet every few hours). Any urine passed will be more concentrated than usual. The tongue and lips will appear to be dry. The skin is less elastic than usual (if you take a small amount of skin on the forearm between the fingers and gently pull the skin up and then let it go, it should spring back; if the child is dehydrated, it will take time to go back). The child will be irritable. The eyes will appear to be sunken, as will the fontanelles in a baby. The child lacks energy and may go into a coma.

If these signs are present, the child must be seen by a doctor urgently for assessment.

Complications

Gastroenteritis can, occasionally, lead to loss of body fluids and important minerals (electrolytes) which can, in turn, lead to convulsions, kidney failure, heart irregularities and even death.

Appendicitis

This is the inflammation of the appendix; the child may become acutely unwell or the onset may be slower. It is rare in babies and relatively rare in young children.

Characteristics

The child:

- may have pain in the abdomen, initially centrally, but later settling on the lower part of the right side
- will have a raised temperature
- will usually have a loss of appetite
- may vomit
- may have a change of bowel habit, either diarrhoea or constipation
- may have bad breath and a dry, coated tongue.

SPECIFIC CARE

The doctor should be consulted, and the child will probably be admitted to hospital for surgical removal of the appendix.

COMPLICATIONS

If treatment is delayed, the appendix may burst and cause peritonitis (inflammation of the membrane lining the cavity of the abdomen).

Infections of the urinary tract

Infections of the urinary tract are common infections seen in children. They occur more in girls than boys.

CHARACTERISTICS

The child:

- may pass urine more often than usual (the urine may be foul smelling)
- may have pain when passing urine
- may have lower abdominal pain
- may have a raised temperature
- may vomit.

An older child may urgently need to pass urine and may, as a result, be incontinent.

SPECIFIC CARE

- The child will need to be seen by a doctor.
- A sample of urine will probably be taken – the carer will be shown how to do this.
- The child may be prescribed antibiotics.
- The temperature will need to be controlled.
- The child will be encouraged to drink plenty of fluids.
- Pain relief, for example paracetamol, may need to be given.

COMPLICATIONS

Untreated repeated urinary tract infections could lead to damage in one or both kidneys and this may result, in severe cases, in kidney failure.

Infections of the blood

Acquired Immunodeficiency Syndrome (AIDS)

This is an illness caused by infection with the human immunodeficiency virus (HIV). The virus damages the immune defence system, leaving it vulnerable to attack by infective organisms.

Note: If a person has been infected with human immunodeficiency virus but her immune system has not been affected, she is HIV positive. This person does not have AIDS, although AIDS is likely to develop at some time in the future.

EFFECTS OF THE VIRUS

Human immunodeficiency virus may enter the body via one of the routes listed below. It then infects the lymphocytes (crucial to the defence against infection). The infected lymphocyte may die, or the virus may lie dormant; if dormant, there may be little or no effect. Sometimes the child may have a mild, flu-like illness and then apparently recover.

The incubation period for the virus is six months to ten years. The virus can be found in blood, semen, breast milk, saliva and urine of infected persons. The following methods of transmission carry a high risk:

- unprotected sex with an infected person
- via blood (either by intravenous drug users sharing contaminated needles or by a transfusion of infected blood or blood products)
- infected tissue donation
- an infected mother can pass the disease to the unborn child *in utero* or via infected breast milk.

HIV FACTS

A child born to an infected mother will probably have HIV antibodies, since these will have been transferred to the child either just before or during birth. This does not necessarily mean that the child is infected, and it may be up to eighteen months before a definite diagnosis can be made.

Since 1985, the testing of blood in the UK has eliminated transmission of the virus via blood transfusion. However, in some parts of the world, testing is not carried out.

Characteristics

The child with AIDS may:

- be prone to infections, including diarrhoea, mouth infections (particularly thrush) and chest infections
- have a fever and night sweats due to the infection
- have enlarged lymph glands
- lose weight
- fail to thrive
- have developmental delay.

Specific Care

There is currently no cure for AIDS, and death may be anticipated eventually. However, treatment can be given to alleviate symptoms, as in any illness; for example, antibiotics for infections and fluid replacement for diarrhoea.

The same principles of care apply to a child with AIDS as with any other sick child. However, at all times particular care must be taken to prevent the spread of the virus to those in contact with the child. When the child is well there should be no reason for her to be kept away from school, playschool or other activities.

Protection of Carers and Others

Day-care establishments and hospitals should have a policy for dealing with body fluids which should be followed at all times. The carer may be looking after a child who is HIV positive without any knowledge to that effect.

This policy would include:

- covering cuts or grazes with a waterproof plaster
- wearing disposable latex gloves when dealing with blood, urine and vomit
- using one per cent hypochlorite solution to cover any blood spillages. The area should then be wiped over with a gloved hand using disposable cloths, which should then be discarded into a bag and sent for incineration. The area should then be washed with hot, soapy water
- washing the hands after dealing with spillages (even if gloves have been used)
- avoiding sharp instruments that could result in injury.

If a carer punctures her skin, and there is a possibility that any body fluid has been in contact with the punctured area, the carer must thoroughly wash the area with soapy water and encourage the puncture to bleed. She must then seek urgent medical advice. An accident form must also be completed.

ACTIVITY

Working in a group, imagine you are working in a day nursery. Write a procedure, 'Dealing with Spillages', for the workplace. Consider, for instance, where you will keep the gloves; if they are kept in a central location, they may not be accessible when needed. Where will you store your one per cent hypochlorite solution? How will you ensure that the discarded material is incinerated? Where will it go whilst waiting for incineration?

Hepatitis

Inflammation of the liver, caused in most cases by one of two viruses.

Type A virus causes hepatitis A (infective hepatitis) which has an incubation period of ten to forty days.

Type B virus causes hepatitis B (serum hepatitis) which has an incubation period of sixty to one hundred and sixty days.

Characteristics

The child may:

- feel tired
- feel generally unwell
- lose her appetite
- have a raised temperature
- be jaundiced
- have dark urine and pale stools.

Hepatitis B can be transmitted in similar ways to HIV. The policy on protection of carers as described for HIV (see opposite page) applies equally to hepatitis B.

Specific Care

- The child will need to be seen by the doctor.
- The child should be cared for at home (or in hospital, if the doctor advises).

- Rest is very important.
- Encourage the child to drink plenty of fluids.
- Scrupulous hygiene is vitally important, as this is an extremely infectious disease. Ideally, the child should be cared for in her own room and she must use only personal towels, which should be kept separate from others. If there is more than one toilet in the house, this should be allocated for the child's personal use; if not, extremely thorough hygienic practices will need to be carried out.

COMPLICATIONS

The child may feel unwell for many months after the infection; once free of infection, she may feel well one day and poorly the next. She may therefore have to return to school/playgroup on a part-time basis.

Hepatitis B can cause death through liver failure.

A number of people who have had hepatitis B remain carriers. A carrier is someone who does not suffer from the infection, but who is capable of passing the infection to others.

Vaccination against hepatitis B is available for people who are particularly at risk, for instance health workers.

Infections of the skin

These can be caused by:

- bacteria, such as impetigo
- viruses, such as warts and verrucas
- fungi, such as ringworm
- insects, such as scabies
- worms, such as toxocara.

Impetigo

Impetigo is an infection of the skin caused by bacteria that most commonly affects the face (although it can affect other parts of the body). It is easily spread by contact with infected flannels and towels.

CHARACTERISTICS

The child may initially have small blisters which break down, leaving weeping areas that crust over.

Specific Care

- It is highly infectious, and the child should therefore be cared for at home.
- Separate face cloths and towels should be used for each member of the family (as always).
- The carer should wash her hands after touching the face.
- The child should be encouraged to leave the crusts alone.
- The child will need to see a doctor, who will usually prescribe antibiotics. She will also advise when the child can start mixing with other children again.

Complications

These are uncommon, but if the condition is untreated, generalised infection may result.

Warts

Warts appear as raised lumps on the surface of the skin. They can occur all over the body and can be spread by direct contact with an infected person.

Warts will eventually disappear, but sometimes treatment is desirable because of pain or unsightliness. Various treatments are available over the counter at chemists, usually in the form of a weak acid. However, these must be used with care, as they may cause the surrounding skin to be burned. If unsuccessful, the wart may be treated by freezing with liquid nitrogen – so-called cryosurgery – but again, some discomfort is almost inevitable, so many doctors may advise a 'wait-and-see' approach.

A verruca is simply a wart that, by virtue of its position on the sole of the foot, has been pushed inwards. Treatment is the same as for warts. It is sometimes recommended that the child wears a rubber sock to prevent the spread of the infection when swimming.

Athlete's Foot

Athlete's foot is a fungal infection that particularly affects the areas between the toes, a habitat in which the fungus thrives. It is infectious and can be transmitted in bathrooms, shower areas and swimming pools. The child will complain of itchy feet, particularly between the toes, where the skin will be found to be pink and flaky. The intense itching – and hence scratching – may lead to bleeding.

The doctor will prescribe treatment, usually in the form of a powder or a cream. If the carer is worried that the condition has not cleared up as expected or that the child's nails have become infected, a doctor should be consulted again.

The carer should carefully wash and dry between the child's toes each day. Ideally, socks should be of cotton material, and shoes made of natural material should be worn. The child should keep the feet covered when walking around the house. Each member of the family should have separate towels.

Ringworm

Ringworm is a fungal infection of the skin, which appears as a red ring. it can also affect the scalp, where it may cause bald patches. The infection can be passed from animals to people, but more usually it passes from person to person. The child will need to be seen by the doctor, who will prescribe treatment.

Prevention of spread is effected by washing hands thoroughly after touching the area and using separate towels and flannels. If the infection came from an animal, it should be taken to a vet for treatment.

Head Lice

The head louse is an insect which lives on the scalp; although it can be seen by the naked eye, it has a tendency to appear the same colour as the hair, making it difficult to find. The adult lays eggs on the shaft of the hair close to the root. These eggs are called nits; they are small, oval-shaped structures, which at first glance look like dandruff. Unlike dandruff, though, they are very firmly attached to the hair.

Once the egg has hatched, the insect bites the scalp and causes intense itching.

The lice can transfer from one head to another very easily by direct contact and they are not choosy about the type of hair they infest. If a child has head lice, treatment should be carried out as soon as possible. The carer should note that treatments change frequently because head lice are masters at developing resistance to treatments, and the health visitor, doctor or pharmacist should therefore be consulted before treating.

Once treated, the louse can no longer cause harm, and the child can return to her usual routine. It is important that members of the same family, or those in close contact with the child, are inspected and treated as necessary.

Prevention of infestation is not easy because of the close proximity in which young children play and work, which allows easy transmission.

However, children should be encouraged to brush their hair thoroughly each day, as this will break the legs of the lice, making it impossible for them to lay their eggs near the base of the hair. The use of conditioner after washing the hair can serve as protection against head lice.

ACTIVITY

You are working in a day nursery. Over the last few weeks, many children have been affected by head lice. You have informed the parents of the affected children and asked them to treat their children. However, you feel that it would be worthwhile to run a teaching session for all parents. You have decided to keep the session short – just fifteen minutes. Write to the Health Education Unit in your area and ask for a copy of any leaflets on the subject; they may also have some teaching materials you could review. The health visitor may have some further information and be pleased to discuss the project with you.

Once you have completed your research, prepare your session. Consider the handouts you might use, any visual aids, such as an overhead projector, posters or perhaps a videotape. Consider when you might run this session to enable as many parents or carers to attend as possible. Consider also the care of the children in the day nursery whilst this session is being run; make sure that enough staff are available to care for the children.

Scabies

Scabies is a condition caused by the skin becoming infested by an insect. This insect burrows into the skin, where it lays its eggs and causes intense itching. A red rash appears around the infected areas. Scabies is transmitted by direct contact.

Scabies is most commonly found between the fingers, but may also be found in the palms, wrists, armpits, soles of the feet and genital area.

The child should be seen by a doctor, who will prescribe treatment. (Treatments can be bought over the counter at chemists, but they may not be suitable for children.) It is usually recommended that the whole family is treated at the same time because of the likelihood of spread to close contacts.

Threadworms

Threadworms are small, white worms that can infest the bowel. Infection occurs when the eggs are ingested. These are usually picked up on hands and will be ingested if the child puts the hands in the mouth. The eggs are very small and can be passed from one person to another via bed linen, towels, clothing or unwashed vegetables and soil.

Threadworms are contagious and easily pass from one person to another. They cause itching around the anus, particularly at night. The child will scratch, eggs will be caught under the nails and the cycle may repeat itself.

Treatment will be prescribed by the doctor. The whole family should be treated at the same time.

Prevention is through meticulous food and personal hygiene, which includes the use of separate towels, scrubbing the nails after a bowel movement and keeping the child's nails short.

Toxocariasis

Toxocariasis is a condition that can occur if the eggs of the toxocara worm are ingested.

The toxocara worm lives in the gut of dogs and cats, and the eggs of the worm are excreted in their faeces. If young children play in an area where dogs and cats have fouled the soil, they may come into contact with the faeces. Young children are particularly at risk because they often put their hands in their mouths and thereby ingest the eggs.

After ingestion, the eggs hatch in the gut and then pass through the intestinal wall. They make their way to the liver and other organs in the body.

This may cause the child to become unwell, with a raised temperature and rash and they feel poorly. As the larvae migrate, they can cause bleeding and infection. In severe infections, inflammation of the optic nerve may occur, and blindness may result.

If there is a suspicion that the child has been in contact with excreta in this way, a doctor should be consulted for advice and tests if appropriate.

Prevention is through public education. All dog and cat owners should regularly worm their animals. Dogs should be prevented from entering children's playgrounds by dog-proof fencing.

ACTIVITY

You have recently been appointed as a nanny. The family has three children under the age of five. They own three cats. You have been asked for advice on worming these cats. Find out from the local veterinary surgery the current recommendations.

Conclusion

Childhood infections range from mild such as the common cold, to severe and even life threatening, such as some types of meningitis. The course the infection takes depends to a large extent on the organism that causes it, but factors such as the child's general health may also have an influence. For these reasons the carer should keep a close eye on the child and be vigilant of any changes in her condition that might suggest seeking a medical opinion.

13

Congenital Factors Affecting Health

A congenital abnormality is present at birth. Congenital abnormalities may occur as a result of inherited factors, as well as a number of other factors which are less clear cut. Infection, medication, cigarette smoking and alcohol intake during pregnancy are examples of known causes of congenital abnormality.

Congenital abnormalities may be identified prenatally, at birth or in the first year of life, when they may be picked up at the child surveillance clinics.

Genetic inheritance

In the nucleus of each cell there are forty-six chromosomes arranged in twenty-three pairs. Half of the chromosomes have come from the mother and half from the father.

Each chromosome has thousands of genes on it, and these carry the information for individual characteristics or development. A gene that controls a specific feature is found in the same place on the same chromosome in each individual.

The individual has two genes for each characteristic; these will usually complement each other, but sometimes one is stronger than the other and is referred to as the dominant gene, the weaker one being referred to as the recessive gene. A relatively straightforward example of dominant and recessive genes is that of eye colour. Brown eye colour is usually a dominant gene and blue eye colour a recessive gene. If both parents have brown eyes, and have inherited two genes for brown eyes from their parents, then all children of these parents will have brown eyes. This is represented in Figure 37.

If both parents have brown eyes and each inherited one dominant brown gene and one recessive blue gene from their parents, of four possible

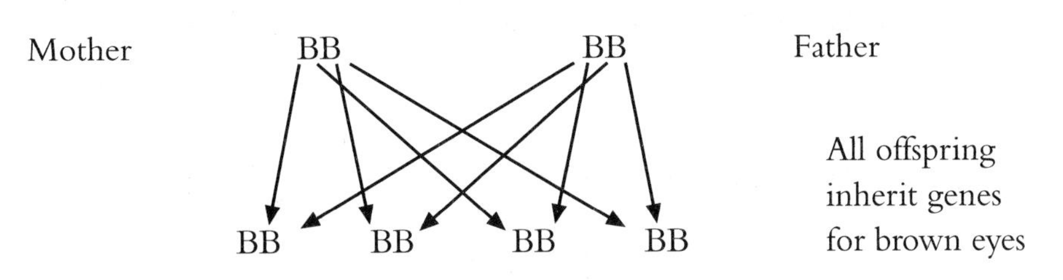

Figure 37 Inheritance (1) Brown eye colour where both parents have brown eyes and have inherited dominant genes

offspring, there is a one in four chance that a child will have brown eyes, having inherited dominant genes from both parents; a one in four chance that a child will have blue eyes, having inherited recessive genes from both parents; and a one in two chance that two children will have brown eyes having inherited one dominant gene and one recessive gene (see Figure 38).

These examples are relatively straightforward; however, they provide a good example of inheritance, which is usually more complex than eye colouring. Of the twenty-three pairs of chromosomes, twenty-two pairs are autosomes (i.e. they have the same functions and have a similar appearance). The twenty-third pair are the sex chromosomes. They are dissimilar and are referred to as the X chromosome and the Y chromosome. A female will have two X chromosomes, and a male will have an X and a Y chromosome.

Some characteristics are inherited through sex-linked inheritance. The X chromosome carries more genes than the Y chromosome, which is smaller. Some diseases, such as haemophilia, can be inherited by a male if the mother is a carrier (i.e. if the mother has inherited the recessive gene for haemophilia from one parent). If he inherits the X chromosome carrying the affected gene, there is no matching gene on the Y chromosome, and the boy will therefore have the disease.

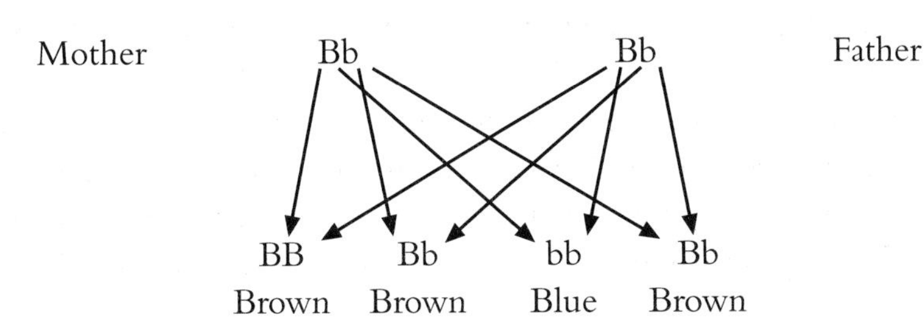

Figure 38 Inheritance (2) Brown/blue eye colour where both parents have brown eyes and have inherited one dominant brown-eye gene and one recessive blue-eye gene. One child has brown eyes (two dominant genes), two children have brown eyes (one dominant gene, one recessive gene), one child has blue eyes (two recessive genes)

Mutations

Mutations can occur. This is when an abnormality is not present in either of the parents, yet the child displays it. Fortunately this is uncommon.

EXTRA CHROMOSOMES

Sometimes a chromosome does not divide properly, and both chromosomes of a pair may end up in the ova or the sperm. Once fertilised, there will be three chromosomes where there should be a pair. This is called trisomy, and an example of this chromosomal defect is Down's syndrome, which is the result of trisomy 21.

Genetic counselling

A couple may be referred to a genetic counsellor:

- if they have an inherited disease
- if there is a member of the family with an inherited disease
- if there is a possibility of one of the couple being a carrier.

The genetic counsellor will discuss the risks of congenital abnormalities that are inherited or familial (run in families).

Abnormalities of dominant genes

Fortunately, this method of inheritance is not very common. An example is Huntington's chorea, but features of this condition are not seen in childhood.

Abnormalities of recessive genes

CYSTIC FIBROSIS

This is the most common genetic disease, affecting one in 2000 births. Approximately one person in twenty carries the abnormal gene.

This condition affects the lungs and the pancreas. The secretions produced are thicker, stickier and contain more salt than usual. In the lungs, this results in small air passages becoming blocked and eventually infected. The child therefore suffers from repeated chest infections.

The child will need physiotherapy at regular intervals during the day. The carer is usually taught to do this. The aim is to loosen the secretions so that they may be coughed up. Antibiotics are prescribed whenever the lungs are infected. Sometimes the repeated chest infections can cause a resistance to blood flow in the lungs, which in turn affects the heart which has to work harder. This can lead to heart failure, and for these children a heart and lung transplant may be needed.

In the pancreas, the secretions prevent the digestive enzymes from working efficiently on food to break it down for absorption. This results in food not being absorbed and eventually to a lack of weight gain and possibly failure to thrive. Fat absorption is a particular problem; fat is needed for energy and for the absorption of some vitamins. Unabsorbed fat leaves the gut in its relatively undigested state, making the stools fatty and offensive.

Pancreatic enzymes must be given so that the food can be absorbed and these are given orally with each meal. The child also needs regular vitamin supplements.

Phenylketonuria

Approximately one in 14,000 babies is affected. This is a disorder in which the baby is unable to metabolise the amino acid (a basic unit of protein) phenylalanine. Failure to do so results in a build-up in the bloodstream. Its accumulation prevents normal development of the brain and central nervous system, causing a learning difficulty. A Guthrie test (a heel prick that allows a small amount of blood to be collected) is routinely done on all babies at seven days old. Babies who are found to have the disorder need to have a dietary restriction of phenylalanine from two weeks of life if it is to be effective in the prevention of learning difficulties.

Sickle Cell Disease

A disorder mainly affecting people of Afro-Caribbean origin (approximately one in 200), although it can be found in people from the Mediterranean, Asia and Middle East. The haemoglobin in the red blood cell forms a sickle shape under certain conditions, which can result in the cells clumping together as they pass through the blood vessels. The blockage of blood (sickle cell crisis) can cause damage, for example to bone. A crisis (when acute symptoms occur) may be brought on by strenuous exercise, infection, dehydration, pregnancy or an anaesthetic and may cause the child to have a fit or become unconscious.

It is uncommon for the child to have any problems before the age of six months.

In a crisis the child may have the following signs or symptoms:

Pain

This is caused by the red blood cells clumping in the blood vessels and blocking them. This pain may be felt in various parts of the body, including the joints, kidneys and intestine.

Anaemia

The red blood cells in the child with sickle cell anaemia have a shorter life span than those of a normal red blood cell. This, coupled with the fact that the red blood cell is more fragile than usual, causes anaemia and the child may feel breathless, tired and giddy as a result.

Jaundice

The child may become jaundiced at times due to the destruction of red blood cells.

There is no cure for sickle cell disease. The child will probably be admitted to hospital in a crisis and she will need reassurance, pain relief and rest, and fluids should be encouraged. Folic acid supplements may be prescribed. Folic acid is needed for red blood cell formation. Infections will be treated. Sometimes a blood transfusion is needed. Remember, carers must be able to recognise warning signs of impending problems and seek medical advice. Warning signs and symptoms include raised temperature, swelling and pain.

A blood test for sickle cell disease or sickle cell trait (where the person is a carrier) will be carried out routinely on all susceptible individuals before an anaesthetic, in pregnancy and if the symptoms are suggestive of sickle cell disease.

Sex-linked inheritance

MUSCULAR DYSTROPHY

Approximately one in 500 males are born in the UK with this disorder. There are a number of variants; of these, Duchenne's is the most common and the most severe and will be considered here.

There may be a history of delayed walking. There is muscle weakness, and the child may have difficulty, for example, in climbing the stairs. He may walk with a wider gait than previously. The weakness is progressive, and the child may have lost his independence by the age of nine or ten. Ultimately the heart and respiratory muscles are affected. The child usually dies during teenage years as a result of respiratory tract infections due to the extreme weakness.

There is no treatment, and care is aimed at prevention of wasting of muscles by physiotherapy and keeping the child comfortable. Consideration will need to be given to conditions at home, and it may be necessary for an occupational therapist to organise some home adaptations to assist the care of the child. The child and parents will need specialist counselling to help them to come to terms with a condition that is progressive and ultimately fatal.

Haemophilia

Approximately one in 10,000 males are born with this condition, in which there is a disorder of clotting due to the absence of factor VIII (haemophilia) or the absence of factor VII (haemophilia B, sometimes referred to as Christmas disease). A blood test for clotting time (which will be prolonged) will confirm the diagnosis.

This is a sex-linked condition where the female is the carrier. An affected male will pass the gene onto his daughters, who will be unaffected by the disease but be carriers of the condition. A female carrier will pass the gene on to some of her sons, who will be affected, and to some of her daughters, who will be carriers. (It is possible for a female to have the condition, but for this to happen, the child would have to have a female carrier mother and a father who is a haemophiliac, so this is very rare.)

An affected child may bruise and bleed more easily when he becomes more mobile and may bleed easily when he cuts his first tooth. The carer will need instructions about specific care. The child should be able to have as normal a childhood as possible, but with the carer trying to avoid harm within reason. Haemophiliac children should wear a Medic-Alert bracelet to alert medical and paramedical staff to the condition in an emergency.

Treatment

Any bleeding will need to be controlled. This may be achieved by the administration of factor VIII, which may sometimes be given by the parents (they will be taught this procedure by the specialists). If the bleeding is not controlled or there is a major bleed, the child will need to be admitted to hospital.

Note: In the UK prior to 1985, blood was not screened for the presence of human immunodeficiency virus (HIV). The result was that the virus could be transmitted via a transfusion of blood or blood products. Tragically, some children and adults were therefore exposed to the virus and some have progressed to develop acquired immunodeficiency syndrome (AIDS) (see page 131). Blood and blood products are now heated to kill off the virus before any blood is used, but this does not always happen abroad, especially in some developing countries.

Kleinfelter's Syndrome

Here, there are three sex chromosomes (XXY) and the child is male. Characteristically, these children have very long legs, may have a learning difficulty and are often sterile as adults.

Turner's Syndrome

Here, there is a single X pattern (XO) and the child is female. Growth is often slow and stunted and there is a web-neck. Ovaries may be absent.

Chromosomal abnormalities

Down's Syndrome

In this condition, there is trisomy of chromosome 21 or translocation (when a small piece of one chromosome becomes attached to another pair and prevents its normal activities). The risk of having a child with Down's syndrome increases in women who are older, rising significantly after the age of thirty-five.

Screening

The risk of Down's syndrome can be assessed by a recently introduced blood test called the Triple test (also known as the Barts or Leeds test). If this shows a high risk, an amniocentesis, which is more specific, would be recommended. Diagnosis is made on the appearance of the child and confirmed by a chromosome analysis. The child will characteristically have slanting eyes (upwards and outwards), a flatter facial profile, low ears and a wide bridge to the nose. Heart defects are often present.

Many of these children will have severe learning difficulties, but all of them will need to be assessed for their educational needs. Down's syndrome children tend to be prone to infections, particularly chest infections, and suffer from a higher than average incidence of heart disease.

ACTIVITY

It is likely that you will be involved in caring for a child with a congenital abnormality at some time in your career.

You are working in a day nursery as a supervisor. When a new child is due to start at the nursery, the parent provides general information and also information on illnesses and medication. Over the next year you will care for:

- a six-month-old child with cystic fibrosis
- a two-year-old with a recently repaired cleft palate
- a four-year-old with sickle cell disease.

Design individual questionnaires that you could give to the parents, asking the questions to enable you to give the best care for the individual children.

Other factors associated with congenital abnormalities

Known factors

Maternal infection can result in:

- adverse placental functioning
- the foetus being attacked by the organism
- infection of the foetus as it passes through the birth canal.

If the infection occurs during the early stages of pregnancy (the first trimester), the risks of abnormalities of the foetus are higher. Infection later on in pregnancy can result in growth retardation.

RUBELLA

If the mother contracts rubella in the first trimester of pregnancy, there is a high risk of congenital abnormality. Organs most commonly affected are the ears, eyes and heart. The baby may be born deaf, blind, have heart malformations or develop learning difficulties and is said to have Congenital Rubella Syndrome.

HIV

The human immunodeficiency virus, which is thought to be responsible for causing AIDS, does cross the placental barrier. The child may be born with

HIV antibodies, but only some of these babies go on to develop AIDS. See page 131.

Herpes Simplex

This is the virus that causes genital herpes. To protect the baby from the disease, an elective caesarean section will be performed.

Medication

Many drugs taken during pregnancy may have an effect on the unborn foetus; for instance, the incidence of cleft palate is higher if the mother is taking steroids. Ideally, the mother should consult a doctor before taking any medication during pregnancy.

Smoking

This has been shown to have an adverse effect on the foetus. Babies born to mothers who smoke are found to be of lower birth weight and are more prone to chest infections, asthma and glue ear.

Alcohol

Women who drink heavily during pregnancy may give birth to a baby with Foetal-Alcohol Syndrome. These children are generally smaller, may have heart defects, have a smaller brain and may have a learning disability.

Drug Addiction

Babies born to mothers who are drug addicts are more likely to be premature and of low birth weight. They are often jittery and generally agitated.

Rhesus Incompatibility

This causes Haemolytic Disease of the Newborn. The majority of people in the UK are rhesus positive. (Rhesus is a sub-group of blood type.) A rhesus-negative mother has no antigens to the rhesus factor in her blood. If the father of the baby is rhesus positive, the baby will be rhesus positive, as the rhesus factor is dominant. There will be no adverse effect to the first child, as the blood of the foetus and the mother do not mix.

However, at birth, a few foetal blood cells leak into the maternal circulation. These contain the rhesus factor, which the maternal circulation regards as foreign and therefore attacks and destroys. This is because the mother produces an antibody to the rhesus factor, called Anti D. This Anti D remains in the maternal circulation. In subsequent pregnancies, these antibodies cross into the foetal circulation and start to destroy the red cells of the foetus where the rhesus factor is found. This will lead to the foetus becoming anaemic. The result of this is that, after birth, there is a large amount of bilirubin (the breakdown product of the destruction of the red blood cells) in the blood. If the bilirubin level rises too high it may affect parts of the brain tissue.

Prevention

This problem can be prevented by identifying all rhesus-negative mothers when they first attend antenatal clinics. Anti D is given by injection after delivery, miscarriage or abortion. This prevents the mother producing her own Anti D. However, the injected Anti D is later recognised by the body as being 'foreign' and is removed from the bloodstream. Thus it has prevented the mother making her own antibodies and is itself removed from the body before any subsequent pregnancies. Therefore the next pregnancy is not a threat from rhesus-factor destruction.

Unknown or multifactorial causes of congenital abnormalities

TALIPES

This occurs in approximately one in 1000 children. Talipes is a condition of unknown cause where there is deformity of the foot, which is twisted. The condition is sometimes referred to as clubfoot. There are several forms of talipes. Often surgical correction is required, although in mild cases, physiotherapy may be effective.

CONGENITAL DISLOCATION OF THE HIP

This is one of the most common congenital defects and occurs in between one in 500 children and one in 1000. Girls are more commonly affected than boys. The condition is more commonly present in breech babies and it occurs more commonly when there is a family history of the condition. It is present when the head of the femur (thigh bone) does not fit into the unusually shallow acetabulum (the cavity in the hipbone into which the femur fits). The cause is unknown, although it is thought that it may have something to do with the maternal hormone levels or possibly the position of the foetus in the uterus. It is usually identified when the newborn is examined; if not, it is often picked up in the child surveillance clinic. Occasionally, it is only noticed when the child starts to walk, and then the condition is more difficult to treat.

In mild cases, abduction (movement away from the midline) of the hip can be achieved by the baby wearing a double nappy. She will not usually need any special care other than the usual changes of nappy. The carer, however, will have double the washing load!

In more severe cases a frog plaster may be needed to keep the hips in abduction. Positioning of the baby/child for feeding and cuddling may take a little ingenuity. When the child is a little older and would usually be using a high chair, some modifications will be needed with safety in mind. She will need to be washed carefully, with particular care to the skin immediately under the plaster where rubbing and soreness can occur. There will be an area of plaster cut out so that the child can pass urine and faeces. This area is protected with a waterproof material so that it can be kept clean. However, the carer will need to follow advice on positioning of nappies for the younger child or positioning the older child on the pot or toilet.

It is difficult to get the child into a pushchair or pram with ease and it is particularly difficult to transport the child in an ordinary car seat. The hospital may have some equipment to lend which may be helpful. It is imperative that the carer follows advice on lifting safely.

Older children may need to have traction applied in order to position the hip joint correctly. Some children may need to have surgery for congenital hip dislocation. These children may or may not have been in a hip plaster.

Remember, the hospital will issue specific written instructions for the care of children in plaster casts, and these should be followed carefully.

ACTIVITY

Prepare a leaflet for carers which gives information on caring for a child with a frog plaster. Include suggestions on modifications of equipment the child would need.

Plan activities for a day for the following children in a frog plaster: a six-month-old baby and a two-year-old child.

CLEFT PALATE AND CLEFT LIP

The child may be born with a cleft palate and/or a cleft (hare) lip. The condition occurs in approximately one in 1000 live births. A cleft palate is a hole or split in the palate, a cleft lip is a split in the lip.

The cause is multifactorial, although there is an increased chance of having a child with the condition if there is a history of cleft palate in the family. Mothers taking steroids during pregnancy also have an increased risk of having a child with a cleft palate.

Deformities such as these are distressing to the parents and family and they will need reassurance that they can be repaired. The baby may have difficulty in feeding. Specially designed teats may help. If there is a large cleft, it may not be possible to breast or bottle feed the baby, in which case the baby is fed with a spoon. Boiled, cooled water may be given after the feed so that curds of milk don't collect around the cleft.

A cleft palate is generally repaired around the age of one to two years and a cleft lip is usually closed earlier.

During this first year, a child with a cleft palate will have been referred to many specialists, including:

- the orthodontist: it is necessary to mould the maxilla (the roof of the mouth) into a well-formed arch
- the audiologist: children with cleft palates may have a hearing loss, which may in part be due to the fact that they tend to have repeated ear infections, as the function of the Eustachian tube (the tube that connects the naso-pharynx with the middle ear) may be impaired
- the speech therapist: the child will see a speech therapist early on, well before she can speak, with the intention of developing good speech patterns
- the plastic surgeon: she will generally co-ordinate the various professionals and then operate on the child at the appropriate time.

Heart Disease

A baby may be born with a malformation of the heart or the blood vessels of the heart. The incidence of congenital heart disease is between eight and ten per 1000 live births. It is a major cause of death in babies in the first year of life.

The cause is unknown; however, if the mother has rubella during the first trimester of pregnancy or if she has drunk large amounts of alcohol during pregnancy, the baby is more likely to have heart disease.

Types of heart disease

Atrial and ventricular septal defects: a 'hole in the heart' between the atria or ventricles. This results in blood shunting from the left side of the heart to the right, which means more blood is being pumped through the lungs. Many will close spontaneously in the first few years of life; some may require surgical closure.

Patent ductus arteriosus: in intra-uterine life, blood bypasses the lungs via the ductus, which closes at birth. Failure to close results in some of the blood flowing from the aorta to the pulmonary artery, and the work of the heart is increased. Sometimes the presence of this defect is not known until the child is three or four years old. Treatment involves heart surgery to tie off the ductus.

Coarctation of the aorta: a narrowing of part of the aorta, which causes a partial obstruction, resulting in a high pressure of blood before the narrowing and a lower pressure after the narrowing. The heart therefore has to work harder to overcome the defect. Surgical treatment may be necessary; the age at which this is done will depend on many factors.

Valve stenosis: the aortic, or mitral, valve may be thickened (stenosed) and will therefore be less efficient. A replacement valve may be needed.

Fallots tetralogy: there are four defects:

- thickening of the pulmonary valve
- ventricular septal defect
- thickening of the right ventricle
- positioning of the aorta over both ventricles.

The baby may become cyanosed (blue) during activity, for example crying. As the child grows, she learns to keep activities in check so that rest periods can be taken. Treatment of the condition depends on the general condition of the child and the age, and will usually involve surgery.

Transposition of the great vessels: the aorta is situated over the right ventricle (not left), and the pulmonary artery is situated over the left ventricle (not the right).

This condition usually results in death unless surgery can be carried out.

The specific care of children with heart abnormalities will depend on the condition and treatment. The parents should be able to give clear instructions on the care needed. Many of these children should be encouraged to have as normal a lifestyle as possible. Some will require regular medication. If surgery is required, the child will usually be admitted prior to surgery for investigations and preoperative care. The parent(s) are encouraged to stay with the child. When the child is discharged, the parents will be given instructions for care.

Spina Bifida

Spina bifida is the malformation of the spinal arch which protects the spinal cord. It occurs in approximately one in 400 births. The disability will vary. Spina bifida occulta is a very mild form of the defect and no specific care is required. Babies with a meningocoele (a sac containing cerebrospinal fluid apparent over the spine) or a meningomyleocoele (a sac containing cerebrospinal fluid and nerve tissue apparent over the spine) will need surgery soon after birth so that the sac can be covered and protected from drying and possible infection. Some of the children will be paralysed, with urinary and bowel problems. The professionals involved in caring for the child will give expert advice on the care of the baby.

Spina bifida may be detected by screening when blood is taken at sixteen weeks of pregnancy to detect the levels of alphafoetoprotein (AFP). A high level may indicate the foetus has spina bifida, and the mother will be offered an anomaly ultrasound scan which will give a detailed picture of the unborn baby. The cause is unknown; however, it is familial (tends to run in families). There is some evidence to suggest that folic acid deficiency may be implicated as the cause, and women are advised to take folic acid supplements prior to getting pregnant and for the first twelve weeks of pregnancy.

Cerebral Palsy

This is a defect of the part of the brain that controls movement or posture. This damage may have happened before birth, during birth or soon after birth. There is no specific cause, although a number of factors may be implicated. These include anoxia (lack of oxygen) before, during or after birth. The child will have some degree of weakness affecting one, two or all limbs.

Cerebral palsy may be identified soon after birth, but is more commonly diagnosed sometime in the first year of life, when the child may be slow at meeting the usual milestones.

The affected muscles may be floppy (flaccid) or stiff (spastic). There may be evidence of learning difficulties.

There is no cure for cerebral palsy, but treatment is aimed at maximising the child's motor and intellectual development. Soon after the condition is diagnosed, the child may be assessed in a paediatric assessment centre, where many specialists, including the paediatrician, psychologist, occupational therapist, physiotherapist, audiologist and speech therapist, will assess her over a period of time. Together with the parents, a plan is made to give the child the best chance of achieving her potential.

The care the child needs will revolve around the outcome of the assessment. It will probably include regular physiotherapy and speech therapy. Schooling will be considered, as will early years education. Some children will need to go to special schools.

Epilepsy

This is a result of a sudden, brief disruption of the normal electrical activity in the brain. It affects between four and six children per 1000. Epilepsy can run in families, may occur as a result of brain injury, either before or during birth, and may be caused by a lack of oxygen, infections or low blood sugar, amongst other things.

Classification of epilepsy can broadly be divided into:

- generalised fits
- generalised absences
- focal, or partial, fits.

GENERALISED FITS (GRAND MAL)

These may occur at any age (although they are uncommon in children less than six months old), during the day or at night, many times a day or very infrequently.

They are characterised by various phases that may include:

- aura: this may precede a fit and may be apparent to the child. The type of auras that occur are very diverse and can include such sensations as a taste in the mouth or a funny smell
- tonic: the body stiffens due to muscle contraction, and the child falls to the ground. Contraction of the laryngeal muscles may produce a characteristic cry

- clonic: uncontrollable jerking of muscles – during this time, the child may be incontinent of urine or faeces and produce excess saliva
- a period of unconsciousness.

This may be followed by a period of sleep, after which the child may be a little disorientated.

Care of the child during a generalised fit

- Ensure that the area is safe. Do not move the child, except to put her in the recovery position (see page 66); stay with the child, loosen any tight clothing, but do not restrain the child. After the fit, make her comfortable, give reassurance and allow the child to sleep or rest.
- If the child has been incontinent, she will need to be washed and given clean clothes. The child may feel acutely embarrassed by this, and the carer will therefore need to be tactful. An older child may wish to see to herself.
- If the child hit herself during the fall, this incident will need to be reported to the parent (and person in charge if in playgroup, etc.) and the accident book would need to be filled in. If the carer suspects that the child has suffered any adverse effects as a result of the fit, medical help should be sought.
- If the fit lasts more than five minutes or if the child goes straight on to another fit, a doctor should be called.

Generalised Absences (petit mal)

These attacks occur in approximately two to five per cent of all epileptics. They are characterised by a brief loss of consciousness, and there is usually no muscle involvement. The onset of the problem is usually between the ages of five and nine and frequently ceases at puberty.

The attacks usually start abruptly. The child may drop an object due to a slight loss of muscle tone, but it is uncommon for the child to fall to the ground. The attacks usually last for a very short time – five to ten seconds – and the child will stare blankly ahead, often blinking or slightly twitching.

These absences are frequently missed or, if seen, put down to lack of concentration. The child can usually follow on with the activity or conversation she was involved with prior to the absence, but may need to be reorientated.

These absences can cause problems with schoolwork if they are frequent, due to the many periods of loss of consciousness. They may also cause problems if the child has an attack whilst swimming or riding a bicycle.

Care of the child during a petit mal fit

- If you suspect a child in your care has petit mal, report your suspicions to the person in charge or to the parent.
- It may be necessary to reorientate a child who has just had an attack, and a gentle reminder should help.
- The child should always be accompanied when swimming, and specific advice may be necessary.

FOCAL OR PARTIAL FITS

These are divided into simple and complex fits. Only part of the brain is affected in this type of epilepsy.

Simple partial fits

Consciousness is not impaired. Fits are characterised by either a sensation – for example, numbness or tingling – or rhythmic twitching or jerking of a limb (or part of a limb).

Complex partial fits

There may be an aura; the child may then appear distracted or confused and repeat a series of movements which serve no purpose, such as lip smacking or plucking at clothes. Sometimes this type of epilepsy may be difficult to detect.

Care of the child during a focal or partial fit

Ensure that the area is safe and talk to the child; often they can still hear and will find this reassuring.

GENERAL INFORMATION

Known epileptics are advised to wear a Medic-Alert bracelet. They do not need to go to hospital unless they do not recover from the fit. Medical assistance would be required for any child not previously known to be epileptic. The carer should inform playgroups, nursery school, schools or clubs that the child is epileptic. At the same time, it is helpful if some information about managing the fit could also be given so that any unnecessary fuss can be avoided.

Fits can usually be controlled by using medication. There are various anti-convulsant drugs available, and the specialist will prescribe the one most suited to the child. It is important that the therapy should be taken as directed. If medication is forgotten, there is a possibility of another fit occurring. There is a tendency for children to improve spontaneously.

Conclusion

This chapter has provided the reader with an insight into some congenital abnormalities and the many factors that can affect the unborn child. Carers may care for a child with a congenital abnormality not included in this section, and they are advised to seek specialist information on the specific condition. This information can often be accessed from libraries or by writing to voluntary associations which are often set up to provide support for families. A list of some of these can be found in Appendix 1, but this is not a definitive list and local libraries often stock books listing various associations.

14

Environmental Factors Affecting Health

The aim of this chapter is to look at several childhood conditions that are affected by the environment. Some children develop an allergy to a substance in the environment, causing conditions such as asthma, eczema or a nut allergy. These are known as external conditions. The internal environment is partly controlled by the endocrine glands which secrete hormones, the underproduction of which may cause diabetes or shortness of stature for example.

Allergies and the allergic reaction

An allergic reaction occurs when a foreign substance, usually a protein, causes the immune system to over-react in a harmful way. This foreign protein is called an **allergen** (or antigen) and it stimulates excessive production of certain types of antibodies.

- An allergic reaction does not usually occur on the first occasion the body is exposed to the allergen, but may occur after a subsequent exposure.
- The foreign substance may be inhaled, ingested or enter via the skin.
- Allergies tend to run in families.

There are many different types of reactions children may have to lots of different allergens. The more common reactions are described below.

- Itching: this may be general or in one particular area.
- Rash: the more common allergic rashes include a nettle rash which is red and the spots are almost joined together, or an urticarial rash which looks like swollen weals.
- Swelling: there may be swelling of the lips, mouth and tongue. **Note:** If this happens emergency action must be taken to keep the airway open (see page 187) and an ambulance should be called.
- Wheezing: the airways may become narrowed, as in asthma, and a wheezing sound may be heard.

- Abdominal symptoms such as discomfort, nausea or vomiting may occur if the child is allergic to a food.

CARE OF THE CHILD

Reassure her by staying with her – if the carer is worried in any way a doctor should be called. If there is any threat to the child's breathing then place her in the recovery position (see page 66) and be ready to start the ABC procedure (see page 187) if necessary. An ambulance should be called.

PREVENTION

If the child develops an allergic reaction to any substance then that substance should be avoided. If there is uncertainty about the allergen then the child may be referred by the general practitioner to a specialist who may perform some tests to ascertain which allergen is implicated.

If the reaction has been serious the specialist might suggest that the child wears a Medic-Alert bracelet which is inscribed with the details of the allergy. It may be that it is recommended that the child carries an 'easy-to-administer' adrenaline injection. This should be taken everywhere with the child. The parents will be taught to use the injection and should ensure that all those who have care of the child know how to use it.

Anaphylactic shock

This is a medical emergency. Anaphylactic shock is a massive allergic reaction to an allergen such as an insect sting, a drug, for example penicillin, or a food such as nuts. Anaphylactic shock can be recognised by:

- rapid swelling in the back of the throat which impairs breathing, or
- unconsciousness.

If the child does not receive urgent attention, death may result.

The child should be injected with the adrenaline she carries around with her as soon as possible. The carer is advised to seek expert tuition in the administration of these drugs if there is a possibility that she might need to use one.

Asthma

Asthma is a condition in which there is intermittent narrowing of the respiratory tubes due to an allergic response. There is often a family history of asthma, eczema or hay fever.

The allergen irritates the cells of the respiratory tract to produce a chemical (histamine), which causes muscle constriction (bronchospasm), swelling and increased mucous secretion. The air passages are therefore considerably narrowed.

As the airways become increasingly narrowed, breathing becomes more difficult. The characteristic wheeze may also be heard as the child breathes out and is sometimes heard when the child breathes in. At least one child in ten is affected by asthma.

CAUSES (SOMETIMES CALLED TRIGGER FACTORS)

Asthma is often associated with an allergic response and can be triggered by:

- exposure to an inhaled antigen, such as pollen, the house dust mite (which lives on shed human skin) or animal fur
- infections, such as the common cold
- exercise
- emotion, excitement or stress
- air pollution – some children are sensitive to cigarette smoke or to fumes from various substances, such as car exhaust
- cold air
- food.

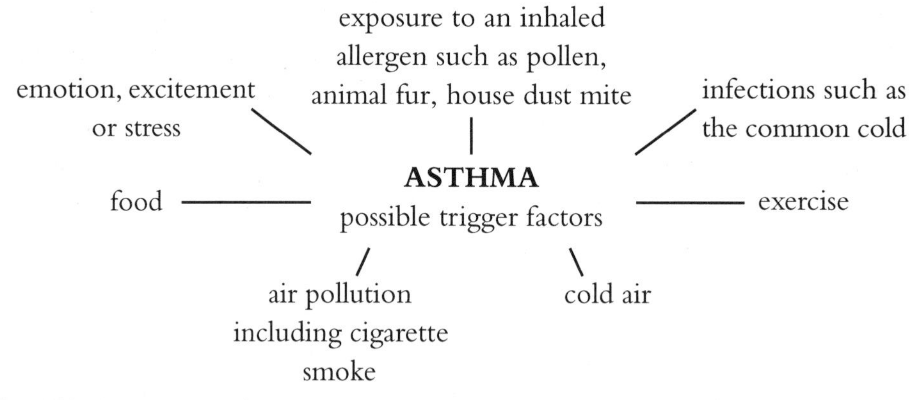

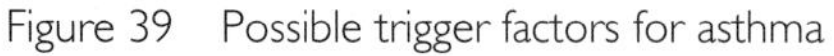

Figure 39 Possible trigger factors for asthma

EFFECTS ON THE CHILD

The onset of an attack may be gradual or abrupt. In general, if the attack is in response to an infection, onset is gradual. If it is in response to an antigen, it will have an acute onset. The child will have a cough, which initially is dry, irritating and unproductive and is characteristically worse at night. Later, the child may cough up and swallow small amounts of thick sticky mucus. The child may become breathless, and the wheeze can be heard as the child breathes out through these narrowed airways. She is often very frightened at this stage and may sweat and appear pale. The older child may sit up, thus making breathing easier.

If the carer looks at the chest at this stage, she may observe that the child is breathing more rapidly than usual and may have some rib recession. The child may have difficulty speaking. A child who has rapid respiration, difficulty speaking and rib recession needs to be seen urgently by a doctor.

Care of the Child

If this is the first episode or if the carer is worried about the child at any stage in the course of the attack, medical help should be requested.

- Stay calm – the child is likely to be anxious.
- Stay with the child, reassure her and avoid fussing.
- Try not to ask too many questions which need responses. The child may be using all available energy for breathing.
- Children often find the sitting position the most comfortable, support with pillows as necessary. A younger child will probably find it more comforting to sit on the carer's lap.

A child who is known to have asthma will usually have treatment with her, which should be given as directed by the parents. If there is little or no response to the treatment, medical advice should be requested. In some cases it may be necessary to telephone for an ambulance. If the child is away from her parents, they should be telephoned and asked to return, because ill children are usually best reassured by their parents. Warm fluids may soothe the throat and help the child feel a little better. Try to distract the child, for example by reading a story. This may decrease the anxiety.

Treatment

Bronchodilator drugs (sometimes called 'relievers') work on the muscles in the airways to open up or dilate them and thus help in the reversal process. Commonly prescribed bronchodilators include Ventolin (Salbutamol) and Bricanyl (Terbutaline). They can be given via an inhaler or orally. Inhalation is the preferred method, as this has the advantage of working directly on the respiratory tract and therefore results in fewer side effects. Recently, 'spacer devices' have been used for children. These have the advantage of enabling the child to inhale the medication without needing the careful co-ordination required by other inhalers. If the bronchodilator is not effective, medical assistance should be requested. The doctor may administer the bronchodilator through a nebuliser. This is a machine that delivers the dose up in a fine mist, which is delivered via a mask.

Steroids may be given in an acute attack. They have powerful anti-inflammatory properties and will complement the bronchodilators. If the child fails to respond to the treatment, she may need to be admitted to hospital. The child will already be frightened and should be kept as calm as possible. Ideally, the carer should stay with her.

Preventative Treatment

This will be considered if the child has frequent or severe episodes of wheezing.

The child may be prescribed:

- Intal (sodium chromoglycate) given via an inhaler; this must be given regularly as directed
- inhaled steroids, for example Becotide
- the doctor may suggest that the child takes a dose of the bronchodilator before exercise, particularly if this is known to cause wheezing.

The child and carer are often asked to measure and record the child's peak flow reading (which indirectly measures the airway narrowing). Readings taken while the child is well will form a basis for the normal reading for that child. During an asthmatic attack, the readings will drop and give the doctor an objective measurement of the severity of the attack. Sometimes the doctor devises an action or care plan for the child. This is organised so that the carer knows what action to take if the peak flow drops and at what stage medical help should be sought.

Eczema

Eczema is characterised by dry, itchy skin – red, rough areas may be seen. It affects up to one in ten children. There are two main types of eczema: atopic eczema and seborrhoeic eczema.

Atopic Eczema

Atopic eczema is the most common type seen in children. There is often a family history of eczema and/or hay fever and asthma.

It is uncommon for a child to develop atopic eczema before the age of three months. Generally, forty per cent of children have grown out of it by the age of two years and ninety per cent by teenage years.

Effects on the Child

The condition is characterised by periods of remissions and relapses. The skin is dry and scaly. When there is a relapse of the condition, there is intense itching, which is worse at night and may cause sleep disturbance. This leads to scratching. The skin becomes red and inflamed. Fluid-filled vesicles may appear on the skin and these tear and weep when scratched. This leads to loss of fluid and the child feels very thirsty. The fluid dries on the skin and forms a crusty exudate. The torn skin can be an entry for infection, which is a frequent complication of eczema. Later, there may be some loss of pigmentation of the skin and it may go on to have a leathery appearance.

Care of the Child and Treatment

Treatment is aimed at decreasing the itching and combating the dryness of the skin; this is usually achieved by the use of moisturising and steroid creams. Moisturising cream should be applied to the body at least twice a day. Several moisturisers may be used; the doctor and carer may have to try several before the best one for the child is found.

- Moisturising creams should be used regularly during the day, for instance aqueous cream or E45 cream.
- Emollients are oily preparations that are soothing to the skin and should be added to the bath water. They are usually prescribed by the doctor. Some need to be dissolved in boiling water before being added to the bath water. Soap should be avoided because it tends to dry the skin and, if perfumed, may itself be an allergen. Soap substitutes include aqueous cream, which is available over the counter at the chemist or on prescription. The bath water should be tepid, never hot, as the heat is an irritant. Sometimes it is advised not to bath the child every day because of the general drying nature of bath water.
- Steroid creams or ointments need to be prescribed by the doctor. (Steroid creams or ointments are anti-inflammatory and they decrease the allergic reaction.) The weakest cream that is effective should be used sparingly. The carer must use them as instructed and must wash her hands after use, as the cream or ointment may be absorbed and cause unwanted effects in the carer. Sometimes the carer is advised to wear protective gloves when applying these creams.
- Antihistamines may be prescribed because of their anti-itch properties and because they are not addictive. They are particularly useful at night

because of their sedative properties, which allow the child to get some sleep.
- Tar preparations are sometimes used for stubborn cases.

GENERAL MANAGEMENT THAT HELPS

- Pure cotton clothing is cool and absorbent.
- Avoid overheating the room – children with eczema feel more comfortable and itch less if they are cared for in cool temperatures. They should avoid direct sunlight and any direct heat.
- Clothes should be washed in non-biological washing powders, and fabric softeners should be avoided.
- Usually no dietary restrictions are necessary, but sometimes a doctor may feel that it is worthwhile trying a special diet, for example, the elimination of milk and milk-based products. This must, however, be tried with the supervision of a dietician.

Sometimes children with skin complaints may be teased by their peers. The carer must be aware of this possibility and deal with any problems.

PREVENTION

There is no known prevention for eczema, but it is recognised that breast feeding a baby up to four to six months is beneficial in the avoidance of allergy.

COMPLICATIONS

Infections of the skin can occur because of the scratching. The child may require antibiotics from the doctor, either as ointments, creams or oral medication. Infections of the skin should be prevented as far as possible by discouraging scratching and ensuring the finger nails are kept clean and short. If the child scratches at night, it may be a good idea to put cotton mitts on the hands at bedtime. It is also a good idea to use cotton pyjamas that fasten together where the top and the bottom part meet.

The condition can put a strain on the whole family if the affected child has disturbed nights. This can cause stress and poor performance at work or at school.

Nut allergy

Whilst it is not known how many children in the UK suffer from peanut allergy, the carer needs to be aware of the potential problem as the numbers are on the increase. It must be remembered that peanuts and other nut products may be found in a large range of foods. If a child is allergic to nuts then it is extremely important to read the list of ingredients contained in products and exclude those that have any nut component from the child's diet. It is also important to remember that removing the nuts from a dish is simply not enough, the offending protein may still be left.

EFFECTS ON THE CHILD

Nut allergy may present in any of the following ways:

- swelling of the lips, throat, tongue and face
- general rash over the whole body
- abdominal pain
- vomiting
- loss of consciousness.

Most children who are allergic to peanuts have an anaphylactic reaction and medical assistance is urgently required (see page 159).

Parents will be given specific advice concerning the child's diet and treatment if there is any reaction. It may be that the child needs to carry an 'easy-to-administer' injection of adrenaline and all carers should be taught how to use the injection.

ACTIVITY

Prepare an information card for student primary school teachers which includes the following information:

- how to deal with an asthmatic attack
- the action of preventers and relievers
- the correct use of inhalers.

ACTIVITY

You are working as a nursery nurse alongside a health visitor. A child aged two-and-a-half has severe eczema. Unfortunately, she has got into the habit of scratching when she is not occupied. The health visitor has asked you to plan activities for the child that will distract her from scratching.

Write up your plan in the form of a report that you will give to the health visitor.

Hormonal deficiencies

The internal environment is, in part, controlled by the endocrine glands which secrete hormones directly into the blood stream. Hormones are chemicals released in one part of the body that have an effect in another part. These endocrine glands can potentially go out of control and either not secrete enough hormone or release too much.

Hormones are secreted from the pituitary gland, the thyroid gland, the parathyroid glands, the adrenal glands and the ovaries or testes and the Islets of Langerhans in the pancreas.

Diabetes

Insulin is a hormone which controls the amount of sugar in the blood. In diabetes there is insufficient insulin produced by the pancreas, resulting in the blood sugar level being higher than normal. There are two types of diabetes. The first is called insulin-dependent diabetes. In this type, the patient requires injections of insulin – this is the type that affects children.

The second type is called non-insulin-dependent diabetes and is controlled by medication and diet, or diet alone. This is more common than the former type, but is not often seen in children.

CAUSE

The cause of diabetes is unknown; however, it does occur more often than might be expected in families (that is, it is familial). It is thought that a viral infection at an earlier stage in life may have acted as a trigger. In the UK, approximately one child in 1000 develops insulin-dependent diabetes.

EFFECTS ON THE CHILD

Sugar needs to be absorbed from the blood in order to be used by the cells. The signs and symptoms of diabetes arise because the sugar in the blood cannot be utilised by the body.

Raised levels of blood sugar lead to:

- sugar in the urine (glycosuria). This occurs because the kidney tubules cannot re-absorb the large quantities of sugar from the urine.

This in turn leads to:

- large amounts of urine being passed (polyuria), causing
- thirst (polydipsia) to compensate for the polyuria.

As the sugar is lost from the body it cannot be used for energy. The body therefore breaks down fat and protein to use as energy. The breakdown of fat and protein leads to weight loss, increased appetite and tiredness. When fats are broken down and used, ketones are released, and these may leave a characteristic smell like pear drops on the child's breath.

Sometimes the condition develops quickly, and the child may become dehydrated due to the polyuria. The child may also lose consciousness.

If diabetes is suspected, a blood test will confirm a raised blood sugar level. Urine testing will usually confirm sugar in the urine and ketones may be present.

CARE OF THE CHILD

The child will be admitted to hospital for the initial treatment and stabilisation of the condition. The care is based on the balance of insulin, diet and exercise.

Insulin

Whilst in hospital, the child will be assessed to determine the amount of insulin she will need. The hormone insulin is injected – it cannot be given orally, because it would be digested before it had an effect.

Hospital staff teach the parents, and the child if she is old enough, to:

- measure the correct amount of insulin. Insulin is prescribed in units, so a special syringe, gun or pen is used
- rotate injection sites to prevent thickening of the tissues. The areas that are used as injection sites include the arms, thighs, buttocks and abdomen (see Figure 40, page 168).
- clean and store insulin syringes (if used)
- store the insulin at the correct temperature in the fridge
- test the blood sugar levels at regular intervals. Note: blood sugar levels should be kept within normal levels, as advised by the doctor, to prevent complications
- test the urine for sugar
- recognise symptoms of high blood sugar levels (hyperglycaemia) and low blood sugar levels (hypoglycaemia).

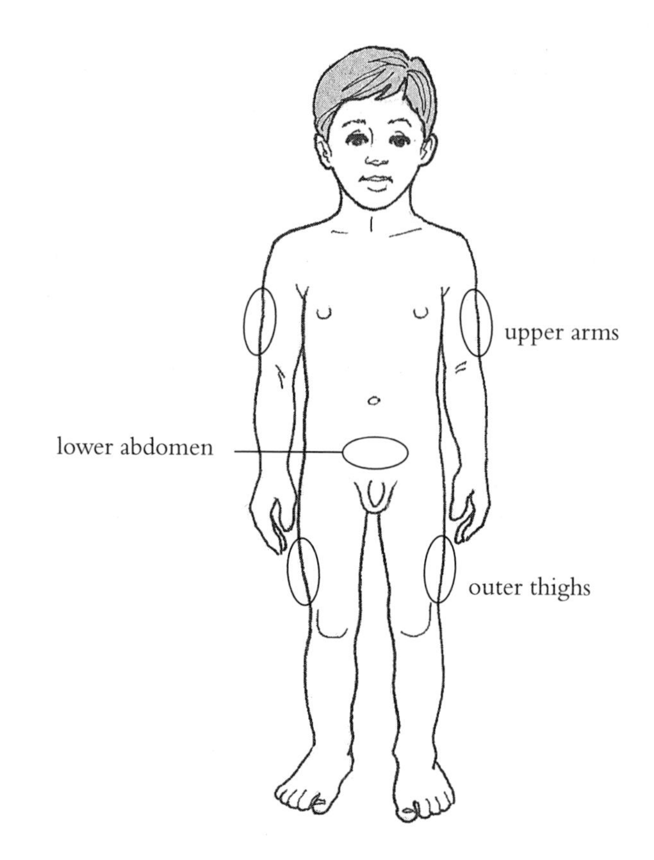

Figure 40 Injection sites for insulin

Diet

A dietician will advise the parents on the importance of providing a well-balanced diet. She will usually suggest that the child is given three meals and three snacks a day. Specific advice is given to families to meet the individual needs.

Exercise

Exercise should not be restricted. However, it may be necessary to take in more food before strenuous exercise. Medical advice should be followed.

HYPOGLYCAEMIA (LOW BLOOD SUGAR)

The causes of hypoglycaemia are:

- too little food
- too much insulin without adequate food intake
- too much exercise without adequate food intake.

Characteristics

The onset is rapid. The child may become increasingly irritable and lack concentration. She may be sweaty and/or dizzy, complain of a headache, vomit and may lapse into unconsciousness.

Treatment

Once these features have been recognised, steps should be taken quickly to reverse the situation. All diabetics are encouraged to carry a sugary snack or drink with them, which should be taken if the child is conscious. If the child has lost consciousness, a doctor and an ambulance should be called, and the situation treated as an emergency.

The child's parents should be informed of all hypoglycaemia attacks. Prolonged hypoglycaemia can cause brain damage, as the brain depends on glucose for normal functioning.

Hyperglycaemia (high blood sugar)

The causes of hyperglycaemia are:

- too little insulin
- illness, such as infections.

Characteristics

Hyperglycaemia attacks are gradual in onset. A child will have the symptoms of thirst, passing large quantities of urine, feeling of drowsiness, breath smelling of pear drops, nausea or vomiting, hot and dry skin. This condition can lead to unconsciousness.

Treatment and First Aid

The parents must be informed.

A conscious child should be given insulin as directed by the doctor and also must be seen *urgently* by a doctor. If the child has lost consciousness the situation must be treated as an emergency. The child's airway should be checked to see that it is clear and then she should be placed in the recovery position and the carer must be prepared to do the ABC routine if necessary. An ambulance should be called by dialling 999. Tell them that the child is in a hyperglycaemic coma. Stay with the child until the ambulance arrives.

Complications

Complications of diabetes other than hyperglycaemia or hypoglycaemia tend to occur later in life. They can be prevented to a large extent by careful management of the condition. The complications are mainly associated with the narrowing of arteries by fatty deposits, which can have an effect on the heart, kidneys, nerves and eyes.

GENERAL INFORMATION

The carer of a diabetic child should:

- be observant for signs of increased thirst, hunger and frequency of passing urine
- seek expert help if the child is unwell because the diabetes may become out of control
- inform the parents if any infection is noted
- inform parents of any problem with eyesight, as diabetics are more prone to sight problems than non-diabetics
- be aware that the sleeping child may be unconscious, particularly if she is sleeping at an unusual time of the day and is sweating, or hot and dry
- *if the job description demands*, be able to test urine and/or blood for sugar content
- build high standards of hygiene into daily care and be more disciplined regarding timing and quantity of meals
- follow the recommended dietary intake
- monitor the amount of exercise taken.

ACTIVITY

Design a leaflet of no more than six sides of A4 paper entitled 'I have diabetes'. It should be aimed at children under seven years old and contain the following information: a definition of diabetes; a description of how the child may have felt before being diagnosed; the treatment and tests; recognition of hypoglycaemia and hyperglycaemia.

The information could be based on a well-known fairy story. The pictures and written work must take into account the child's age and expected stage of development.

Growth deficiency

The pituitary gland controls many of the other endocrine glands. It also secretes growth hormone which, if there are deficient amounts, will lead to growth stunting.

There are many causes of growth deficiency, and the child will be referred for assessment and treated with injections of growth hormone if necessary.

Hypothyroidism

The thyroid gland secretes thyroxine. Low levels of thyroxine cause hypothyroidism. The condition is routinely screened for, seven days after birth when the Guthrie test is taken. Treatment prevents stunting of mental and physical growth.

Conclusion

This chapter has looked at some of the common and less common conditions that are seen in children as a result of the environment in which they live. It is very likely that the carer will have responsibility for a child who suffers from asthma at some time during her career, and it is important that she is familiar with the care and treatment necessary both as a preventative measure and for treating an asthmatic attack. Similarly it is also likely that she will care for a child who suffers from eczema. Other conditions discussed in this chapter are less common but the vigilant carer may well be the person who observes slight changes suggestive of a condition which requires medical attention.

15

Hospitalisation

Each year approximately one million children are admitted to hospital in the UK.

In most hospitals, children are cared for on children's (paediatric) wards where the parents are usually welcome to stay. Visiting times are unrestricted, so that even if the parents cannot stay, they are welcome at any time.

Parents are encouraged to care for the child as much as possible, thus reducing the child's anxiety at what can be a stressful time. Hospitalisation can be distressing. Much of the preparation and care given to young children is aimed at trying to reduce this distress.

Emotional reaction to hospitalisation

Psychologist John Bowlby, who studied the effects upon young children relating to attachment and subsequent loss of their parent, and James and Joyce Robertson, who made a series of films entitled *Young Children in Brief Separation*, outlined three phases of attachment and loss reactions in young children.

Protest

The child will cry and cling to the parent in an attempt to prevent them leaving. She will become very distressed when the parent leaves and may cry uncontrollably.

Despair

The child realises that the parent is not going to return. She is inconsolable, but eventually appears to settle in. However, she is often quiet, uncommunicative and appears sad and may regress. The child becomes upset and angry when visited.

Detachment

The child 'settles down'; she accepts the situation and may show indifference to the parent on return. This stage is seen less commonly than the other stages, but may be reached if the child has been in hospital for a long time and has been cared for by many different carers. She will appear to be happy, but is trying to ignore the hurt of losing her parents.

Note: it is important that anyone caring for a child who is in hospital or going into hospital is aware of these stages and understands them so that the child can be cared for sensitively and that steps can be taken to avoid separation if possible.

The effects of these reactions can leave the parents distressed and the child totally bewildered by the whole experience. In the past, many children took a long time to overcome the effects of hospitalisation, suffering nightmares and anxiety.

As a result of the work on separation by Bowlby and Robertson, the Platt report (1959) was published to encourage the nurses of sick children to care for their psychological as well as physical needs. One recommendation was that provision should be made for mothers of children under five to stay with their child. Later, the voluntary agency National Association for the Welfare of Children in Hospital (now called Action for the Sick Child) was set up to 'raise awareness of the emotional needs of all sick children'. The reaction children show to hospitalisation depends on their age, stage of development, past experiences and parental influences.

Factors that may affect a child's reaction to hospitalisation

AGE AND STAGE OF DEVELOPMENT

Birth to six months

A baby will generally have been cared for on a one-to-one basis. She will be affected by the changes caused by hospitalisation. The parents are usually encouraged to stay in the hospital with the child and to care for her as much as possible to provide security.

Six months to two-and-a-half years

The child between these ages has a relatively limited vocabulary and is not yet able to understand all that is said. She will have built up a firm relationship with the carer and is often distressed by separation. Separation anxiety is more apparent at this stage, and the child will often protest loudly. She is also affected by changes in routine and regression is common.

It is important that the carer should stay with the child if possible; if it does prove impossible, then she should be encouraged to make full use of open visiting.

Two-and-a-half to four years

Separation anxiety is still a feature in this age group and may manifest itself in the child being excessively clingy, refusing to eat, having sleep problems or withdrawing. Many children of this age see illness as some sort of punishment, and if adequate preparation is not given, worries and anxieties are more apparent.

It is recommended that the carer stays with the child. The child has built up a trust in her, she will be able to offer simple explanations, using language that the child understands. Honesty must be used at all times, because the child will lose trust in the carer if she is misled. The young child may fear separation from parents more than the operation or treatment.

School age

Most children in this age group are capable of understanding a simple explanation of why they need to be hospitalised, but frequently worry that they are missing something important. It is a good idea if the carer stays with the child, although depending on the nature of the admission and the individual child, it may be acceptable to both if full use is made of unrestricted visiting.

Past Experiences of Hospital

The child may have some first-hand experience of hospitals, perhaps through visiting a relative. This experience may be negative or positive, and it may help to discuss 'the time you visited . . . in hospital'; this may provide a forum for the child to express worries.

The initial impression of the hospital is often what will be remembered, and it is therefore important that the carers should strive to make that experience as positive as possible.

If the child has been told that if she behaves in a certain bad way she will be 'taken to the hospital', hospitals may be perceived as places to fear.

Parental Influences

Parents are the best people to prepare children for hospital. They therefore need to be adequately prepared themselves and should be aware of:

- the importance of their presence when the child is in hospital and their role
- what will happen to the child whilst she is in hospital
- the nature of separation anxiety
- ways in which the child might react in order to cope with the anxiety
- the need for kindness and honesty
- the knowledge that their anxiety may increase the child's anxiety.

A child who has some experience of being away from the family for short times may have positive or negative memories of the experience, and these will influence the ability to cope.

Children who are insecure are likely to find hospitalisation more stressful.

Preparation for admission to hospital

Children will be admitted to hospital either as an emergency or planned admission. The amount of preparation that can be done with a child admitted in an emergency will be limited. However, children who have some preparation are less frightened than those who have none. Rodin (1983) stated that children who are prepared for hospital and medical procedures cope better than those not prepared.

A recent recommendation from the report from the Department of Health on the Welfare of Children and Young People in Hospital (1991) states that:

> **Children should, (therefore) be admitted to hospital as in-patients only if appropriate care cannot be provided daily in the community.**

Whether for in-patients or otherwise, paediatric wards and departments should provide an environment which is conducive to the promotion of health and the lessening of stress, with both emotional and clinical health needs receiving constant attention.

POINTS FOR CONSIDERATION

The child may be:

- frightened of the unknown
- frightened by stories she might have heard about hospitals
- worried about being away from her family (however, parents should be made aware that there are facilities for them to stay with the child and that these may be available at no extra cost)

- worried about how to behave
- frightened about the loss of her independence
- wary of strangers
- worried about the food she might be expected to eat
- worried that she will be in pain
- worried that she may be left in hospital (particularly relevant if the child is not visited often).

PREPARATION

Leaflets

Hospitals often send out leaflets or a booklet to the parents to share with the child some weeks before she is due to be admitted. Although the hospital sends these out early, it is a good idea to delay sharing them with the child until about a week before the admittance date. The leaflets or booklet will usually contain information about the ward, such as:

- things to bring into hospital
- mealtimes
- facilities for parents to stay
- the role of parents when the child is in hospital
- school
- play and the playroom
- saying goodbye (even if parents are staying in hospital with the child, they will need at least a short break)
- safety
- doctors' ward rounds
- what happens after the child goes home.

Books and toys

Children love to be read to and they will be able to gain information about hospital by listening to books being read. Libraries usually have a good selection of books on the subject of children in hospital. Toys can also be used effectively in the preparation. Fuzzy-felt hospital allows the child to make up hospital scenes and can be used particularly effectively with young children, as can Playmobil hospital, and of course, dolls and teddies.

Pre-admission visits

Increasingly, hospitals are offering pre-admission visits for children due to be admitted in the near future. The child, parents and any siblings are invited to come into the hospital to meet members of staff and to see the ward for themselves. They are given a tour of the ward, shown the beds and the lockers, the toilets, the playroom and the toys. They are also shown some of the equipment that is commonly found on a children's ward, such as a stethoscope. The Rogue's Gallery is pointed out to the children and their families (see page 83). These visits are usually arranged for a Saturday as it is usually more convenient for the family. Children often spend some time in the playroom playing with the toys and meeting the play specialist.

Preparation in the early years setting (playgroup, nursery school and school)

Many experts feel that preparation for hospital should be included in pre-school and school activities, thus allowing the children to gain positive images which will encourage them to talk and play, thereby acting out their worries. It is important that any questions about hospitals should be answered honestly and in language appropriate to the child's understanding.

Preparation the day before admission

Allow the child to be involved in packing the things she will need in hospital. The booklet will probably give a list of things the child will need. It will include:

- a sponge bag (containing a sponge or flannel, a toothbrush and toothpaste, soap, talcum powder (if used), comb or brush)
- towels
- clothes (she will probably be dressed for most of the day)
- night clothes
- slippers and shoes (some hospitals have an outside play area)
- a few favourite toys, books or tapes (ideally these should be named)
- a comforter if one is used (again, this should be named)
- a favourite drink and some non-perishable food (check with the nurse in charge)
- family photographs to put on the bedside table
- nappies (if appropriate)
- special bottles or feeders
- the Personal Child Health Record (see page 26)
- books and magazines for the child and the parents.

Tell the child what will happen. Use language that she will understand. Always tell the truth, and if you don't know something, say so, but promise that you will find out when you arrive. If a carer is going to stay, tell the child – it will reassure her that someone familiar will stay. If no one can stay, tell the child how often someone will visit. Answer the child's questions – she will often want to know a lot of different things about being in hospital.

THE DAY OF ADMISSION

It is a good idea to keep the routine as near to normal as possible. If the child is going in for surgery as a day case, the parents may have been told not to give the child anything to eat or drink after a certain time. It is very important to adhere to these instructions, and if the child is old enough to understand, then she should be told. However, with a younger child, it may be a case of organising the rest of the family to eat earlier or later than usual, so that the child doesn't see the food.

When the child arrives on the ward, one of the nurses will already be allocated to organise the child's care and will greet her. The nurse will introduce herself by the first name (this helps keep the situation as informal as possible), talk to the child and thus start to build up a rapport. The child will be shown her bed, introduced to other children and told where her parent will sleep (if staying). The nurse will then take the parent and child to find some toys to play with whilst the child is formally admitted to the ward. The nurse will then gather information about the child by talking to the child and parent so that an individual care plan can be drawn up.

General information, including name (and any pet name), age, date of birth, next-of-kin (including family unit), siblings, immunisations to date, religion and special cultural practices, will be gathered either before admission or at this stage.

On admission, the parents are asked about the child's past medical history, including any admissions to hospital. They will be asked what they (and the child) understand the reason for admission to be, so that any misunderstandings can be clarified if necessary. Any allergies and medications the child is taking will be noted.

The carer (and child, if appropriate) will then be asked for information on the child's usual routine. The nurse also needs to find out the following specific information.

Communication

A child's ability to communicate will vary according to the age, stage of development and, to some extent, the personality of the child. The nurse will find out what is normal for the individual and if the child requires any communication aids, such as a hearing aid or glasses.

Hygiene

The nurse will need to establish the usual routine, which includes bathing, washing and cleaning teeth.

Rest and sleep

The child's usual pattern of naps and sleep will be noted and will include information on where the child sleeps, the usual sleeping position and any bedtime routines.

Comfort

Many children have comfort habits, and these often become important during stressful situations such as hospitalisation.

Food and drink

The nurse will need to find out if the child is bottle fed, breast fed or weaned. She will also need to find out whether an older child can feed herself. Any dietary restrictions will be noted.

Play and activity

This will depend on the age and stage of development and includes information on the child's mobility. Any favourite toys or games will be noted.

Elimination

The nurse will need to establish if the child wears nappies, whether she is toilet trained, any special words that she may use and the child's level of independence. The nurse will also need to find out the child's normal bowel habits.

The care plan

Having gathered the information, the nurse, together with the parents, will write a care plan for the child. At this stage, the role of the parents will also be discussed, and the nurse will find out if the parents are going to stay with the child.

Note: the older child (aged five or over) will be expected to attend school on the ward each day (providing she is considered well enough).

IMPLEMENTATION

The care plan will be put into operation and changes or alterations will be made as necessary.

EVALUATION

The plan is evaluated, and reassessment made as necessary.

Soon after admission, the child will be examined by one of the doctors and some investigations may be requested. These will be explained to the child and the parents. Other professionals may now meet the child, depending on the nature of the reasons for admission.

The importance of play for the sick child

Play is essential for all children for physical, intellectual, social and emotional development. It allows them to learn about the world, learn new skills, get on with others and act out fears and fantasies. It remains an essential part of the day, even when they are unwell. Children may be able to come to terms with their illness more easily if they are allowed to play and act out their feelings. Play is an ideal medium through which children learn to cope with stress.

Sick children usually regress and prefer to play with toys that they discarded some time ago. These toys require less concentration and are therefore more enjoyable for children while they are unwell.

Specialist play workers are employed in most hospitals and are in overall charge of play in the ward. Most hospitals have a playroom on the children's ward, and the children have access to painting, sand, water, dough and cooking, as well as puzzles and books. There are usually televisions and video recorders on the ward, and they are increasingly equipped with computers. Some hospitals also have some sort of outdoor play facility.

Hospital play can:

- facilitate communication between children and the professionals
- be used to help in the preparation of children for specific procedures
- allow children to act out any fears and anxieties
- take children's minds off the situation and, since children play as part of their daily routine, help to restore some of the normal aspects of life
- speed recovery, possibly due to decreased anxiety.

The hospital corner in the playroom can provide children with the opportunity to act out fears and anxieties. This corner will need the following equipment:

- syringes (no needles)
- bandages
- masks
- stethoscopes
- bed
- dressing-up clothes
- dolls and teddies.

The play specialist may be involved in preparing children for the following procedures:

- surgery
- intravenous infusion
- change of dressing
- X-ray
- physiotherapy
- removal of sutures.

The specialist will talk the child through the procedure with the aid of photographs and equipment. The child may be encouraged to try on a mask and then look at herself, play with the stethoscope and listen to her own heart sounds (easily heard, even through a toy stethoscope). Other equipment will be made available as necessary.

Play is part of a normal day to the child, so that, by playing, some sort of normality remains in the child's life during this very stressful time.

When providing play facilities, the carer must consider:

- the mobility of the child
- the age and developmental stage of the child, taking into account regression
- use of suitable materials, for example, sand is not really suitable for a child wearing a plaster cast
- that she may need to be the partner in a game
- that a hospital corner is invaluable in a playroom
- that some children are isolated because of their condition, and the play specialist is a very important visitor who may help to relieve the boredom.

MOBILITY

Mobile patients can take themselves to the playroom; immobile patients can be wheeled to the playroom in a bed. With preparation, the bed can be protected in such a way that children can paint, use modelling clay and participate in other messy play. Mirrors can be positioned so that reading in bed is easier, and for patients who cannot turn the pages, a page turner can be attached to the book rest.

AGE AND DEVELOPMENTAL STAGE

Sick children will often find that their concentration span is shorter than usual, and, as already seen, children do regress when unwell. Toys designed for a younger age group which require less concentration are better.

THE PLAY SPECIALIST IN THE INTENSIVE THERAPY UNIT

Children in the Intensive Therapy Unit may be critically ill, but they may still benefit from some sort of play.

Unconscious children will often be able to hear (hearing is the last sense to be affected when a person becomes unconscious), and listening to music or having a favourite book read will be reassuring to them. Any carer involved in looking after unconscious children should always remember that many of these children can still hear and that it is always important to tell them what you are going to do before doing it so that they are aware of what is happening.

Children who are very unwell but not unconscious will often enjoy looking at mobiles or perhaps a poster placed where they can easily see it (this may be on the ceiling). They can listen to a book being read, or to music.

As children improve, they may be ready for more active play sessions. The play specialist may work with the other professionals, for example the physiotherapist, so that activities involve play and thus will be more enjoyable for the child.

It is important to realise that play in such situations should be for short periods, as children may tire easily after the stimulation.

The child admitted to hospital as an emergency

The child admitted to hospital without some of the preparation discussed above may be more anxious and will therefore need some special attention. The nurses, play specialist and others involved in the child's care should be made aware of the situation and will need to explain everything to the child and her parents. However, the same principles of care apply, whether the child is admitted as an emergency or as a planned admission.

Preparation for returning home

When children are considered ready to be discharged from hospital, a meeting should be set up with their parents so that a suitable time can be arranged. Research has shown that, when people are stressed, they do not retain all that is said to them; instructions about medication and care will therefore need to be written down. Parents should also be given telephone contact numbers in case they are worried.

Parents will need to be told that some children do display some disturbance after being in hospital. However, this is less of a problem if they have stayed in the hospital with the child or if the child has been in hospital for only a short time. Children who do react to the stay in hospital may show signs of one or more of the following.

REGRESSION

The child may want to be cuddled more than usual; may wet herself when she has previously been dry or may revert to a more babyish way of speaking. This behaviour will usually last for only a short time, and parents are best encouraged to go along with it. The child needs the parents' time and reassurance.

AGGRESSION

The child is responding to the frustration of being in hospital, and any aggressive behaviour should only last a short time.

SLEEP DISTURBANCE

Some children may want to sleep in the same room as their parents after being in hospital, because they are anxious after their hospital stay. Some children will have dreams or nightmares, which will gradually lessen as they gain confidence again.

PROBLEMS IN SCHOOL

The child's teacher should be made aware of the possibility that these may occur so that she can show understanding.

It is important that parents are made aware of these possible reactions to hospitalisation so that they can respond positively and considerately to the child, knowing that she will overcome them.

ACTIVITY

Prepare a leaflet (no more than two sides of A4 paper) that could be sent out to parents before the pre-admission visit. Include in your leaflet all the information that you think would be beneficial to parents to enable them to help prepare the child for hospital.

Conclusion

Many children are admitted to hospital each year, and many more are taken either to the accident and emergency department or to the out-patient department. For some of these children the experience can be traumatic. However, if the child is prepared for the possibility of being taken to hospital, the traumatic effects can be considerably lessened. It is recommended to prepare the child in an early years setting where discussion, play and the sharing of experiences can take place and any worries discussed.

16 Accidents

An accident is an unpremeditated event resulting in recognisable damage (World Health Organisation).

An accident is something that happens unexpectedly. Accidents are the most common cause of death in children between the ages of one and fourteen and are also the cause of many disabilities.

Children are naturally curious about their environment and are prone to accidents because of their inexperience and their ever-increasing mobility and manipulative skills. Carers have a responsibility to ensure the safety of children as far as is possible and in order to do this they require a thorough understanding of normal growth and development. They will then be prepared for the possibilities associated with the age and stage of development and will be able to provide the necessary protection.

Prevention of accidents

The carer should:

- 'think safety'
- try to see the world through the eyes of children and anticipate potential accidents
- be aware of safety aspects in the children's environment (this may require some initial training by parents or the person in charge, followed by regular updating)
- take opportunities to teach children in their care about safety
- take opportunities to discuss safety issues with other carers
- check equipment regularly – look for any equipment that has been damaged, and check new equipment for the relevant safety symbol
- plan the play layout with safety in mind
- store equipment safely
- ensure the children's clothes are safe

- see themselves as role models. Children observe adults and will often take their lead from them. All the carers' actions should have safety in mind, for example, if cycling a helmet should be worn along with reflective clothing, if driving the seat belt should be worn and all passengers should be appropriately restrained.

Accidents in the early years setting

All accidents in the early years setting must, under Health and Safety Regulations, be recorded in an accident book. The following information must be included:

- full name, address and occupation of the injured person
- date and time of the accident
- place where the accident occurred
- cause and nature of the injury
- name and address of the person who discovered the accident.

Accident books must be kept for a period of three years.

All fatal accidents and major injuries must be reported immediately to the relevant enforcing authority.

First aid

The reader should note that this section aims to provide a brief guide to first aid. The author strongly recommends that any carer working with children should attend a recognised first-aid course.

First aid is the help given to a casualty before the arrival of the ambulance or a doctor. The aims of first aid are to:

- preserve life
- prevent deterioration
- promote recovery.

The first aider must *assess* the situation in which she finds the casualty, as follows.

1 Look out for **danger**, either to herself or further danger to the child. If there are suggestions that the situation is unsafe then steps must be taken to ensure the safety of both. For example, if the carer finds the child lying on the floor holding an electric wire it is possible the child has received

an electric shock. It is very important that the child is removed from the supply before the carer attempts to help as the electric current will give her a shock as well. This can be achieved by knocking the wire away using an object that does not conduct electricity, such as a wooden broom handle or a rolled up newspaper. If there has been a road traffic accident, the traffic should be diverted away from the accident if possible. Although ideally the first aider should not move the casualty, it may be necessary to ensure the safety of both people.

2 Once the situation has been rendered safe the child should be assessed for **response**. It is important to ascertain whether or not the child is conscious. This can usually be done by talking to the child or gently shaking her if there is no response. If there is no response the child can be presumed unconscious and thus will require urgent medical attention.

3 Check the **airway** (**A**). To clear the airway place the child flat on her back, open the mouth and remove any obvious obstructions. Gently tilt the head backwards by placing one hand on the forehead and one finger under the chin. This will ensure that the airway does not become obstructed by the tongue.

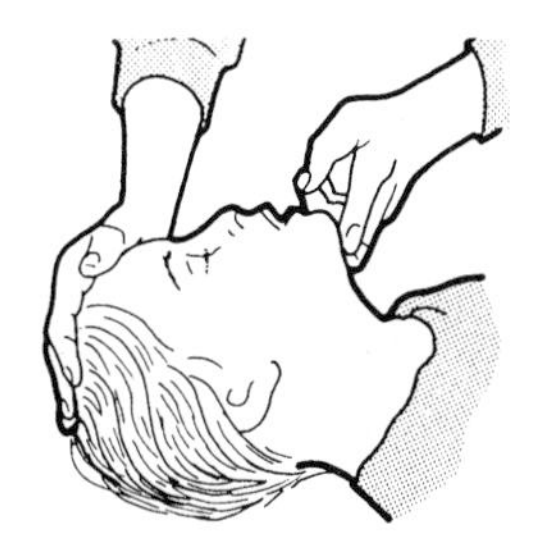

Figure 41 To clear the airway, tilt the head backwards by placing one hand on the forehead and one finger under the chin

4 Check for **breathing** (**B**). Place your head on one side close to the child's face and listen and feel for breathing. At the same time look at the chest for signs of breathing and place one hand on the chest to feel for evidence of breathing. If no breathing is apparent after ten seconds it can be assumed that the child is not breathing and mouth to mouth resuscitation will need to be carried out: *five* inflations, mouth to nose (three seconds per breath).

5 Check for **circulation** (**C**). In a baby, lightly press your fingers towards the bone on the inside of the upper arm you should be able to feel a pulse (brachial pulse) see Figure 42 on next page.

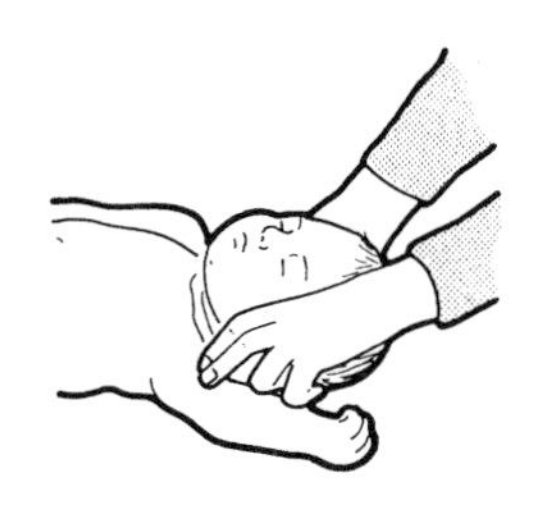

Figure 42 How to find a baby's pulse

In a child, find the carotid pulse by feeling in the hollow between the Adam's apple and the muscle running down the side of the neck.

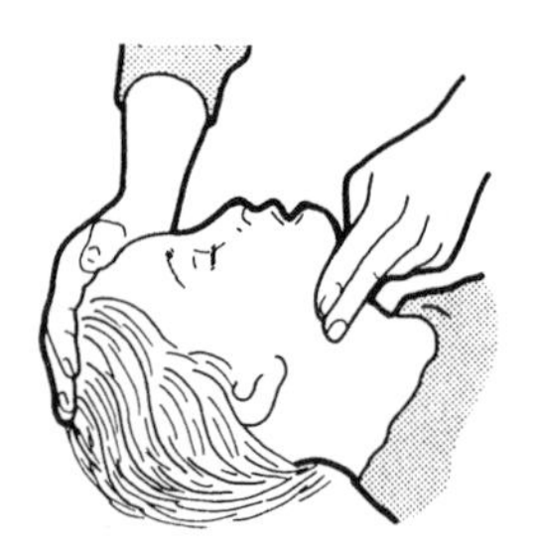

Figure 43 How to find a child's pulse

If a pulse cannot be felt after five seconds it can be assumed that the heart is not beating and there will be no oxygen circulating in the body. It is vital that the first aider commences cardio-pulmonary resuscitation as damage to the brain will occur within a matter of minutes if it is without oxygen.

Resuscitation for babies

Once this assessment has been completed the first aider should be familiar with the correct procedure that needs to be administered.

IF THE BABY IS NOT BREATHING BUT THERE IS A PULSE PRESENT

If help is available, shout and ask someone to phone 999. Ask them to report back to you when they have done so.

You will have started mouth to nose resuscitation. Continue this:

- seal your lips around the baby's mouth and nose and blow gently into the lungs until the chest rises at a rate of approximately twenty breaths per minute. As you blow air into the lungs watch to ensure that only enough air to inflate them is blown in. Take your mouth away to allow the baby to breathe out. Then repeat the procedure.
- Do this for one minute then check the pulse (see above).

If you are on your own perform the procedure above and then carry the baby with you to the phone and dial 999 for an ambulance. In either case you should now:

- **continue mouth to nose resuscitation until the ambulance arrives, checking for a pulse every minute.**

If the Baby is Not Breathing and There is No Pulse

If help is available shout and ask someone to phone 999. Ask them to report back to you when they have done so.

You will have started mouth to nose resuscitation. Continue with cardio-pulmonary resuscitation:

- **find the position where the ribs meet and measure one finger above this point. Once you have found this point use two fingers and gently press down to a depth of 2 cm ($\frac{3}{4}$") at a rate of 100 compressions per minute. After five compressions gently blow into the lungs once (see above). Continue this cycle for one minute.**

If you are on your own perform the procedure above and then carry the baby to the phone and dial 999 for an ambulance. In either case you should now:

- **continue resuscitation, checking for a pulse every minute until the ambulance arrives.**

If There is a Pulse Present and the Baby is Breathing

- **Lay her in the recovery position (see page 66) and dial 999 for an ambulance. Check the pulse and breathing every minute and be ready to commence resuscitation.**
- **Check the baby for any possible reasons for her unconscious state, such as swelling on the head that might suggest a head injury or bleeding.**

Resuscitation for children

If the Child is Not Breathing but There is a Pulse Present

If help is available, shout and ask someone to phone 999. Ask them to report back to you when they have done so.

You will have started mouth to mouth resuscitation:

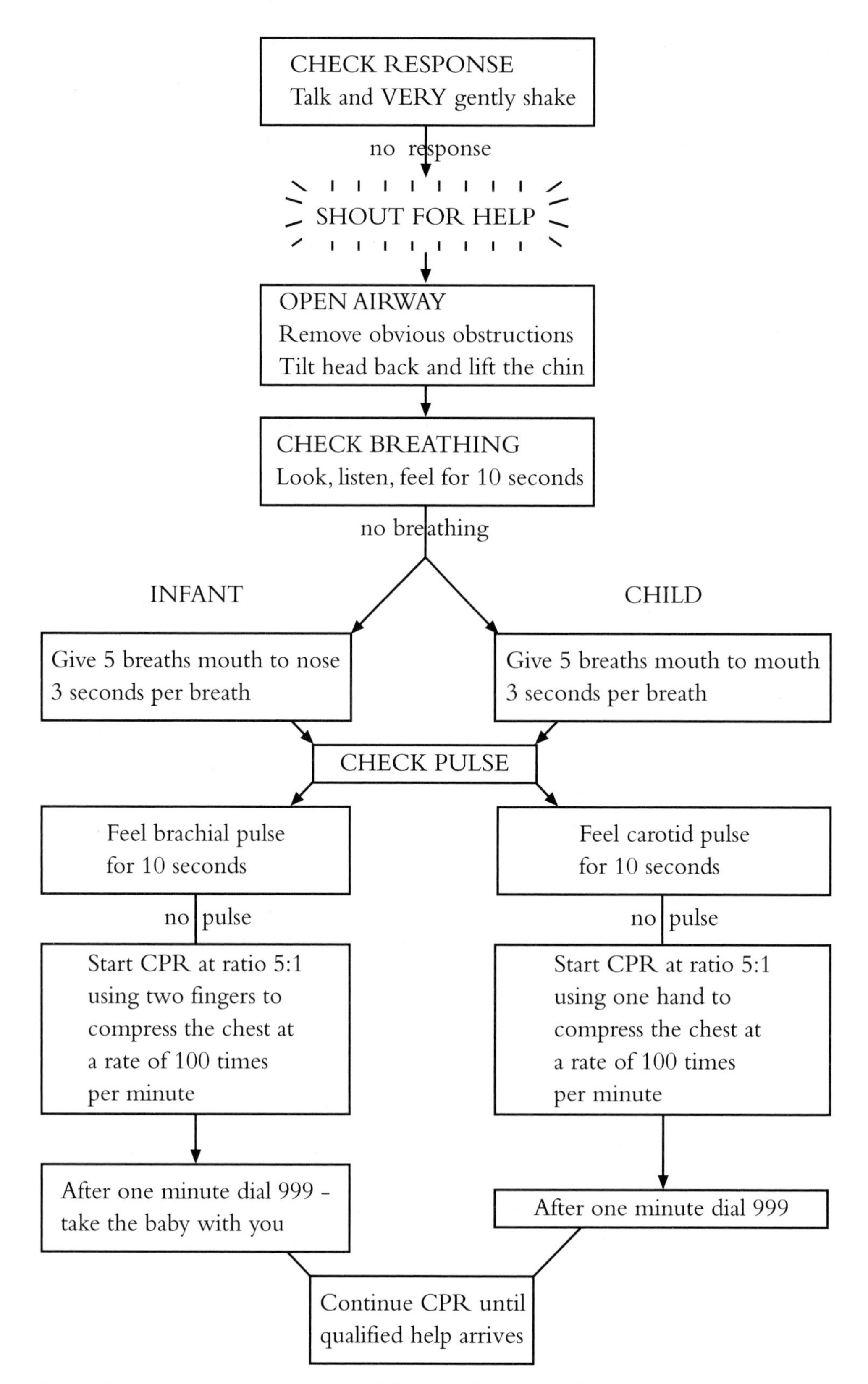

Figure 44 Cardio-pulmonary resuscitation (CPR) procedure – infant/child

- Pinch the child's nose and take a deep breath. Seal the child's mouth with your mouth and blow gently into the lungs until the chest rises at a rate of approximately twenty breaths per minute. As you blow air into the lungs watch to ensure that only enough air to inflate them is blown in. Take your mouth away to allow the child to breathe out. Then repeat the procedure.
- Do this for one minute then check the pulse (see above).

If you are on your own perform the procedure above then leave the child and phone 999 for an ambulance. In either case you should now:

- return and commence mouth to mouth resuscitation until the ambulance arrives, checking for a pulse every minute.

IF THE CHILD IS NOT BREATHING AND THERE IS NO PULSE

If help is available, shout and ask someone to phone 999. Ask them to report back to you when they have done so.

You will have started mouth to mouth resuscitation. Continue with cardio-pulmonary resuscitation:

- Find the position where the ribs meet and measure one finger above this point. In this position use one hand and firmly press down to a depth of 3 cm ($1\frac{1}{4}$") at a rate of 100 compressions per minute. After five compressions gently blow into the lungs once (see above). Continue this cycle for one minute. Check for a pulse every minute and if it is not present repeat this cycle.

If you are on your own leave the child and phone 999 for an ambulance. On return continue resuscitation, checking for a pulse every minute until help arrives.

IF THE CHILD IS UNCONSCIOUS BUT A PULSE IS PRESENT AND THE CHILD IS BREATHING

- Lay her in the recovery position (see page 66) and dial 999 for an ambulance. Check pulse and breathing every minute and be ready to commence resuscitation.
- Check the child for any possible reasons for her unconscious state such as swelling on the head that might suggest a head injury or bleeding.

Head injury

Children seem to bump their heads rather a lot in the early years. This is probably due to their increasing curiosity and mobility. Most of these bumps are minor and require little more than a gentle rub, reassurance and a cuddle. However, it is important that the carer is alert to the possibility of a more serious head injury and knows the action to take.

The danger of head injuries is that they may have caused damage to the brain.

If a child sustains a head injury and the carer is worried *for any reason* then she should seek advice from the general practitioner. The early years worker should inform the parent and if the injury took place in the nursery or school, then an accident form must be completed.

ACTION TO BE TAKEN FOR A HEAD INJURY

If any of the following signs or symptoms occur during the twenty-four hours after the head injury is sustained, medical advice should be sought urgently:

- unconsciousness, even if it is for a short time, or if the child is very drowsy – there is no need to keep the child awake for twenty-four hours. If she sleeps then she should be checked regularly for a normal response when spoken to or gently roused
- headache
- visual disturbance such as double or blurred vision
- vomiting or feeling nauseated
- fits or spasms of the hands or face
- discharge from the nose or ear.

If the child loses consciousness then the airway, breathing, circulation (ABC) routine (see page 187) must be followed.

ACTIVITY

Design a series of leaflets with your colleagues that can be used by all child carers. The titles of the leaflets are:

Prevention of Head Injuries in the Home 0–6 months
6–18 months
18 months to 5 years

Prevention of Head Injuries Outside	0–6 months 6–18 months 18 months to 5 years
Prevention of Head Injuries	in Cars on Bicycles in the Supermarket

Bleeding

Children fall over and sustain small cuts and grazes relatively often. Most of these are minor and require little more than cleaning up and reassurance. The carer must be aware of the importance of prevention of infection and all carers should wear gloves when dealing with cuts. The wound should be cleaned with cool water and a dressing applied if necessary. If the injury happens in the nursery or school then a record of the incident should be recorded in the accident book.

If the child has a severe bleed then the carer must:

- summon medical help
- try to stop the bleeding
- contact the parents.

ACTION TO BE TAKEN IF THE CHILD HAS A SEVERE BLEED

- Wear gloves.
- Sit or lay the child down.
- Apply direct pressure to the wound using a dressing. If none is available use whatever absorbent material is available such as a clean tea-towel.
- Elevate the area if possible.
- Apply a dressing. If the blood soaks through apply another one on top of the first.
- Reassure the child and keep her warm.
- Give her nothing to eat or drink.

If the child loses consciousness then the ABC routine must be followed.

Burns and scalds

A burn is caused by hot dry heat, whereas a scald is caused by something hot

ACTIVITY

List the contents of the first-aid box. What equipment do you have at your disposal if a child does have a severe bleed. Discuss this with your supervisor. Find out who the first aiders in the workplace are and ask them to show you the accident book.

---

and wet, such as steam or liquids. Chemicals, electric shocks and the sun can also cause burns.

If the child sustains a minor burn the area should be placed in a bowl of cold water for ten minutes or until the pain eases. The area should then be covered with a dressing.

If the burn is larger than a two-pence piece, medical assistance should be sought.

ACTION TO BE TAKEN FOR A BURN OR SCALD

- Cool the area. It may be necessary to pour water over the area.
- Reassure the child.
- For larger burns, cover the area with a single layer of cling film loosely applied and seek medical assistance as soon as possible. When using cling film, children should be supervised at all times.
- Do not burst blisters or apply ointments or creams.

If the child loses consciousness then the ABC routine must be followed.

ACTIVITY

On the first day of each work experience find out the position of:

- the fire fighting equipment
- fire exits
- the telephone
- the first-aid kit.

Fractures

A child may have fractured a bone if there is:

- loss of movement
- swelling around the damaged bone

- deformity – the area might look odd
- pain
- tenderness over the affected area.

If the carer suspects there is a fracture the child will need to be taken to the accident and emergency department of the local hospital for an X-ray.

Action to be Taken if There is a Possible Fracture

- The child should be made as comfortable as possible – an arm may be placed into a sling or an older child may be happy to hold it. A leg could be gently tied to the other leg to act as a splint.
- Reassure the child.
- Take her to hospital – two adults should accompany her because there is always the possibility that the child might lose consciousness.
- The child should not be allowed anything to eat or drink.

If the child loses consciousness then the ABC routine must be followed.

Conclusion

It cannot be emphasised enough that any carer could one day find herself in a position where she could save the life of a child if she only knew what to do. Enrol on a first-aid course now!

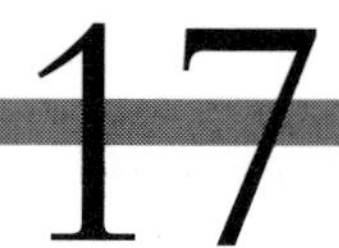

Childhood Cancers

Many different types of cells make up the body, each of which has a role to play in its smooth running. These cells will multiply at the correct rate for the individual to ensure that:

- growth takes place until such time as the adult size has been reached
- old or worn-out cells are replaced.

Cell division is usually carefully controlled. However, if continuous and unrestrained cell division occurs, abnormal cells are formed which crowd out normal cells and cause damage.

This over-production of cells results in a growth referred to as the **primary growth** or **tumour**, and the cells do not function as they should. Some tumours are non-malignant (benign), others are malignant (cancerous). Benign tumours may need to be removed by surgery.

Malignant tumours (cancers) can affect the functioning of cells around them. Some of the malignant cells may break off and spread to another part of the body, usually by the bloodstream or by the lymphatic system. These are referred to as **secondary growths** or **metastases**. Metastases can destroy the function of the cells they invade.

Types of cancer

There are many different types of cancer, just as there are many different types of cells. They are classified according to the cell and tissue type from which they originate.

The most common types of childhood cancers are leukaemias, cancers of the brain and lymphomas.

Causes of childhood cancers

The cause of most childhood cancers is unknown. However, there is some evidence that ionising radiation, viruses and genetic factors may play a part in the causation of some cancers.

Unfortunately, since very little is known about the causes of childhood cancers, little can be done to prevent them. However, carers should keep themselves up to date with information on any research that may identify causes in the future.

Diagnosis

Medical opinion should be requested if the child shows any of the following signs:

- has been excessively tired
- appears pale
- has lost weight
- has been generally unwell for some time
- has developed a lump or lumps that may warrant medical evaluation.

Sometimes signs or symptoms may be picked up in the child surveillance clinic.

If cancer is a possible diagnosis, the child is usually referred to a regional centre for that type of childhood cancer.

Treatment

At present, there are three main types of therapy that are used in the treatment of cancer. These are:

- surgery
- chemotherapy
- radiation.

Surgery

The aim of surgery is to remove the cancer so that the function of the body can be restored and spread prevented. Surgery is most successful for cancers that are limited to an area and have not spread. It may also be used as a palliative measure (alleviates the symptoms but does not cure the disease) when the cancer is causing symptoms that cannot be easily controlled by other means. Surgery may be followed by radiation and/or chemotherapy treatment.

Chemotherapy

Chemotherapy is the treatment of disease by drugs. There are a number of drugs that can be used to destroy the cancer cells. They do, however, have some effect on normal tissue. They are used particularly in cancers that are widespread, such as leukaemia. Chemotherapy may involve the use of cytotoxic drugs. These work by destroying abnormal cells in the body and are particularly effective against the rapidly dividing cells which include cancer cells. Unfortunately, they may also destroy other rapidly dividing cells, such as those in the gut, the hair and in the bone marrow where blood cells are produced.

UNWANTED SIDE EFFECTS OF CHEMOTHERAPY

The unwanted effects include hair loss, diarrhoea, vomiting and anaemia. The child is also prone to infections, because the cytotoxic therapy can destroy the production of white blood cells in the bone marrow. Antibiotic therapy, either as treatment of infection or prophylactically (as a prevention against infection) may be given.

Radiotherapy

Radiotherapy is used in the treatment of cancer to cause the death of cells or a decrease in the growth of abnormal cells. It may be used to shrink the size of the cancer, thus relieving the symptoms, and it can be used as a curative treatment. The dosage of radiotherapy is carefully calculated to minimise damage to surrounding tissue. It is sometimes given after surgery to destroy any remaining cancer cells.

UNWANTED SIDE EFFECTS OF RADIOTHERAPY

The child may be excessively tired after treatment and may feel nauseated or actually vomit. There may be loss of hair from areas that have been treated. Sometimes the skin around the treated area is red and sore. The carer will be given specific instructions on the care of this area.

Leukaemia

Leukaemia is the commonest type of cancer seen in children. It occurs when the bone marrow produces too many white blood cells, many of which are immature and abnormal and therefore do not function properly. (White blood cells help the body to fight infection. There are different types of white blood cells with slightly different functions.)

Leukaemia is defined according to:

- the type of white cell affected
- the onset of the illness – whether it is acute or chronic.

In children, acute leukaemias are more common than chronic leukaemias. Acute leukaemias have a sudden onset, chronic leukaemias have a slower onset and take time to develop.

Cause

The cause is unknown; however, there are several factors that might be involved.

- Radiation – children of mothers who received abdominal X-rays during pregnancy have a slightly higher risk of developing leukaemia.
- Viruses – research has shown that leukaemia may be the result of an abnormal response to a viral infection.
- Chemicals – some chemicals cause leukaemia.
- Congenital factors – there is an increased incidence of leukaemia in children with Down's syndrome.

The effects of leukaemia on the child

The over-production of immature white blood cells results in other blood cells (red blood cells and platelets) being under-produced. This in turn leads to:

- anaemia – this results from a decrease in the number of red blood cells. The child will be tired and may be breathless, pale and generally listless
- bruising and bleeding – this results from a decrease in the number of platelets which are needed for blood clotting. The child will bruise easily and may bleed from her gums when cleaning her teeth. She will also be prone to nose bleeds.

The over-production of immature white blood cells also leaves the child prone to infections and this will lead to:

- raised temperature – the child will feel hot and uncomfortable
- a decrease in appetite which may lead to weight loss
- swollen glands (see page 49). This is an attempt by the body to respond to the infection
- localised pain caused by the infection.

The child may also complain of pain in her bones; this is because the white cells are produced in the bones.

The effects for chronic leukaemia are similar but they are slower in onset.

Diagnosis

This is made after the child has been seen by a doctor, a blood test taken and the increased numbers of white cells and decreased numbers of red cells and platelets are noted. The child will be referred to a regional centre for confirmation of the diagnosis made by a bone biopsy (when a small amount of bone marrow is taken and examined).

Treatment

The aim of treatment is to destroy the abnormal cells. This is hopefully achieved by the use of chemotherapy and sometimes radiotherapy. The child will need several courses of treatment which may be continued over a long time. When the blood test shows no evidence of the immature cells, the child is said to be in remission. However, the treatment is usually continued after this time, because there is a chance of a further relapse.

Sometimes a bone marrow transplant may be performed when the child is in remission. Bone marrow transplants are only possible if a suitable donor can be found.

The survival rates for children with leukaemia have improved tremendously over recent years owing to improvements in treatment.

Tumours of the nervous system

The nervous system is made up of the brain, spinal cord and the peripheral nerves. Cancers of the nervous system cause the highest number of cancer deaths in children after leukaemias. They are the commonest type of solid tumour (abnormal cells that are in one clump). Cancers of the nervous system arise from various areas in the system.

Brain tumours

These cancers can be primary or secondary growths and are uncommonly seen in children under the age of two years. The effects of a tumour in the brain is related to the space occupied by it, causing pressure on other areas of the brain. The following signs and symptoms may be seen – but remember not all are necessarily seen:

- headache – characteristically worse in the morning
- nausea and vomiting – caused by the increased pressure
- visual defects, such as double vision, squints or nystagmus (involuntary rolling of the eyes)
- hearing defects
- muscle weakness
- ataxia or a lack of co-ordination (if the tumour is pressing on the cerebellum – the area at the base of the brain)
- fits – which may be generalised or partial
- decreased appetite causing weight loss.

The child will be seen by a doctor who will carry out a thorough examination and then refer her to a regional centre for further investigations. These include a skull X-ray, a CAT (computerised axial tomography) scan and perhaps magnetic imaging. An EEG (electroencephalogram) may be requested to see if the electrical impulses across the brain have been affected.

TREATMENT

This will depend on the nature and size of the growth. It may be possible for the neurosurgeon to remove the growth completely if it is well defined and in an accessible place. In some cases, radiotherapy may be used to shrink the growth, and this is used particularly if the growth is invasive and inaccessible for removal. The effectiveness of treatment depends on many variables: the size, accessibility, type of growth and whether or not it has invaded other structures. There may be complete recovery, some disability or, in some cases, the treatment may be unsuccessful.

Tumours of the urinary tract

The most common cancer of the urinary tract is a Wilm's tumour, also known as a nephroblastoma. The cause is unknown. There is an increased incidence among siblings and identical twins, which suggests a genetic tendency.

The effects of Wilm's tumour

The carer may notice or feel a swelling in the child's abdomen, commonly at bathtime. It may also be picked up when the child is being routinely examined for an illness. Some children may pass blood in their urine. There may be other general symptoms of malignancy, such as weight loss.

Diagnosis

Abdominal X-rays will reveal a growth, and other investigations will then be carried out to confirm the diagnosis. Tests are also carried out to ascertain the presence or otherwise of metastases (secondary growths which have spread from the main cancer).

Treatment

The child will have the growth surgically removed, either completely or as much as possible. This is followed by radiotherapy and chemotherapy. The survival rates for children with Wilm's tumours are the highest of all the childhood cancers.

Lymphomas

These are solid growths that arise in the lymphoid tissue, mainly the lymph nodes and the spleen. They are subdivided into Hodgkin's lymphomas and non-Hodgkin's lymphomas.

Effects

The child will have enlarged lymph glands. She may have a raised temperature and night sweats (when the child sweats excessively at night, so much so that she may wake and will need to be washed and have a change of clothing). The child will be more prone to infections than usual and may be anaemic. Nausea and vomiting may also be a problem.

Diagnosis

Several tests may be carried out, including taking a biopsy of the lymph gland. Blood is taken and examined, X-rays and scans are carried out, so that an accurate assessment can be made of how advanced the illness is.

Treatment

This usually involves radiotherapy and chemotherapy. Generally, Hodgkin's disease can be treated successfully in childhood.

Bone cancers

Bone cancers are uncommon in children.

Effects

The child will complain of pain over the affected site. There may be evidence of a lump, which is painful.

Diagnosis

This is usually confirmed by X-rays and scans.

Treatment

This may include surgery to amputate the affected limb, and chemotherapy.

Skin cancer

Children rarely develop skin cancer, but the carer needs to be aware of the measures needed to prevent its development in later adult life.

Role of the carer in the prevention of skin cancer

- Keep children out of the sun when it is at its most intense (between 11.00 am and 3.00 pm), ideally longer. Carers should therefore plan the day around these times.
- The child should be dressed in a cotton dress or T-shirt (ideally one with a collar), shorts and a floppy hat.
- Sunscreen (factor 15 or above) should be worn whenever the child is exposed to the sun and should be reapplied after swimming.
- If children need to be outside when the sun is intense, they should make use of the shade.

ACTIVITY

Design a life-size cut-out of a nursery-aged child that will stand up in the nursery, then draw some underwear on the cut-out. Design and cut out a range of clothes and hats that can be attached easily to the cut-out. You are now ready to play a 'safety in the sun' game with the children. You will need to give them some information on sun safety first. Divide the group into small teams and ask them to dress the cut-out according to the weather forecast you describe.

Caring for children with cancer

The long-term outlook for children with cancer has improved over the last decade and it is important to have a positive outlook if at all possible. Children should maintain their usual routine wherever it is feasible.

The effect on the child and the family

THE CHILD

The child's understanding of the illness will depend on several factors including her age, developmental stage and the effect of the illness. She may have to go through a lot of trauma during the diagnosis and treatment. Much of this time may be spent in hospital, which in itself can be a difficult experience. The treatment may have unwanted side-effects, some of which will make the child feel wretched, for example vomiting, or may affect the child's appearance, for example hair loss. The individual care plan must take into account the effect of treatment and include information for the child on dealing with the unwanted effects. The child may be affected emotionally: unwanted effects can lead to fear and anxiety about further treatment; long-term hospitalisation will decrease contact with friends and family. An older child may worry about relapses.

Education

The child will be absent from school or pre-school during treatment of recovery. Liaison between the family and the teachers is essential so that the child can return with the minimum fuss. Teachers or carers will usually keep in touch with an ill child and often encourage the class to write. Sometimes the teachers may approach the parents to ask if they might give an explanation to the other children who may be unduly worried about their fellow pupil. Any explanation offered must always have parental consent and if given, a simplified resumé should be given to the other children. It is important to give some explanation particularly if the appearance of the ill child has changed, such as hair loss after chemotherapy, to avoid teasing.

During the acute phase when the child is in hospital, the hospital teachers will liaise with the child's own teacher, so that the child can keep up when she feels well again. On return to school or pre-school activities, teachers and carers must be vigilant for outbreaks of chickenpox or measles as these conditions can be very severe in children with cancer. If an outbreak occurs the parents must be informed urgently so that the child can be given temporary immunity by the doctor. The family will have been through a traumatic time and they might appear over protective and anxious and it is helpful if the teacher or carer is supportive.

THE FAMILY

The family will probably be devastated by the diagnosis: they may go through a range of emotions including shock, denial and guilt. It is therefore important that they receive support from professionals and they may gain support from one or more of the many voluntary organisations. A social worker may be appointed to support the family and to help liaise between the hospital staff and the family.

A senior doctor will tell the parents the diagnosis and explain the disease process, the treatment available and the prognosis to them. Experience will allow the doctor to judge just how much information to give at one time. The family will be given a phone number as a contact point for questions. Leaflets and books are also made available.

The parents will need to tell other people involved in the child's life of the diagnosis, so that they are aware of the situation. It is important that siblings are given time to discuss anxieties and worries. They may have feelings of guilt because of arguments and disagreements they have had in the past. They may also be affected by the long periods of absence when their brother or sister is in hospital. They may be looked after by a succession of carers, which in turn may result in them feeling left out.

ACTIVITY

You are working in a reception class as a classroom assistant. A five-year-old child has recently been admitted to hospital for treatment of leukaemia. The teacher has discussed with you the idea of writing to the child, with each child in the class contributing. You are aware that their written skills are limited. Draw a spider diagram to give an overview of how you might plan the session. Consider what you will tell the class members about the child in hospital (this would need to be considered with the child's parents, the class teacher and yourself), what activities each member might be able to contribute, and your role in the activity.

Conclusion

This chapter has provided information on many of the childhood cancers. However, it must be emphasised that if the carer is involved in the care of a child with cancer, she should ask the parents for any specific information in order to care for the individual.

18

Terminal Illness and Care

A child is said to have a terminal illness when treatment no longer has any prospect of curing the disease. Death will ultimately result.

The medical team involved will offer help and support to prepare the parents for the eventual death. The aim is for the child to die with dignity. At all times, a very high standard of care is given to make the child as comfortable and happy as possible. The place of death will depend to a large extent on the wishes of the family and the child, and this may be at home, in a hospice or in hospital.

A child may die:

- as a result of a congenital abnormality that is incompatible with life
- unexpectedly, for example as a result of cot death
- suddenly, for example as the result of an accident in the home or a road traffic accident
- as a result of an acute illness, such as meningitis
- as a result of a prolonged illness, for example cancer.

Caring for the child in hospital

A child may die in hospital if she is too ill to go home. The parents and sometimes siblings may be offered accommodation either on the ward or nearby.

The parents will be encouraged to be with their child during the last weeks or days. They will be able to give the child much of her daily care, with the professionals giving treatment as necessary. The parents will be able to take breaks at any time, and help and support will be offered.

Caring for the child at home

Parents will sometimes request that the child be brought home to be cared for by them. This will be discussed with the doctors, and if it is felt possible, the parents will be given every support from the doctor and other members of the Primary Health Care team. Facilities are available for pain or symptom relief to be given. In some areas, there may be a children's hospice which will offer respite care.

Caring for the child in a hospice

A hospice provides care for the terminally ill and for children with life-threatening illnesses which may not be imminently terminal. The hospice may be attached to a hospital. The care offered is personalised care, and more attention than usual can be given to each child. The hospice will often provide respite care, which may be essential because parents can become exhausted providing twenty-four-hour care for the child.

Wherever the child is cared for, carers are encouraged to allow siblings and other children close to a dying child to help in her care. Siblings are usually aware that something is wrong, and it is often better to involve them in doing something positive so that they feel that they helped in some way.

Carers should be honest with children and tell them the situation in language that they understand. They should be allowed to express their thoughts and feelings with the adult, who should accept their reaction (which may be unexpected). However, questions will often come later. Comfort should be natural; children can comfort adults just as adults can comfort children.

If at all possible, the parents will be called to be with the child if it is thought that death is imminent. Unless the child dies unexpectedly, the parents will have been prepared to some extent. However, prepared or not, the moment of death usually comes as a great shock.

Bereavement

After death has occurred, the parents should be allowed to stay with the child and to hold and talk to her and to each other. This is a time to say goodbye and should not be hurried. Later, they may wish to wash and dress the child for the last time.

Grief

Adults and children may go through various stages of grief: some individuals react immediately and some reactions are delayed.

Initially, there may be denial and shock, as the bereaved have not yet accepted the fact of death. The funeral is the opportunity for people to say final goodbyes, and this may enable the family to start accepting that death has occurred. Feelings may be a mixture of anger, guilt, anxiety and depression. Siblings may be clingy during this phase. The grieving phase may be thought of as being over when the situation has been accepted without extremes of feelings.

Support after a child has died

The family doctor will usually visit the family on several occasions to offer support and counselling. The health visitor may also visit several times. Sometimes, the children's ward or the hospice offer self-help support groups for parents and/or siblings. If there are any problems associated with siblings or parents coming to terms with the death, the family may be referred to specialist counsellors.

Cot death (Sudden Infant Death Syndrome – SIDS)

'Cot death' is the term applied to the sudden unexplained and unexpected death of an infant. Most cot deaths occur between the ages of twenty-eight days and one year and it occurs in approximately one per 500 infants; the cause is unknown. However, as a result of epidemiological studies, various risk factors have been identified:

- the sleeping position of the baby (there is a higher incidence of cot death in babies who sleep on their fronts)
- the temperature of the room (the baby should not be allowed to get too warm)
- cigarette smoke (infants who are exposed to cigarette smoke before and after birth are at higher risk)
- method of feeding (breast feeding has been suggested as having a lower risk for cot death, however the evidence is inconsistent).

Cot death is more common in winter, and boys are affected more often than girls. It is more common in:

- babies born to parents in lower social classes
- babies born to young mothers
- babies who have lots of siblings
- premature babies
- babies of low birth weight
- babies of multiple births.

Reducing the Risk

Sleeping position

Babies should be put down to sleep on their back. There is no evidence to suggest that they might vomit and inhale in this position.

There are some exceptions, and these will be advised by the doctor (they include babies with gastro-oesophageal reflux (backward flow of stomach contents) and others with specific airway obstructions).

Smoking

Mothers are advised not to smoke during pregnancy as it increases the risk of cot death. Babies should not be exposed to cigarette smoke. Ideally there should be a ban on smoking in the house and babies should be kept away from smoky atmospheres.

Temperature

Overheating the baby increases the risk of cot death. Babies can get too hot if they are covered with too many bedclothes, if they are dressed in too many clothes or if the room temperature is too warm.

The carer can check the temperature of the baby by placing a hand on the baby's abdomen, which should feel neither too warm nor too cold. Bedclothes are best kept to lightweight blankets. Duvets should not be used, and it is recommended that the baby is placed in the 'feet to foot' position (see Figure 45).

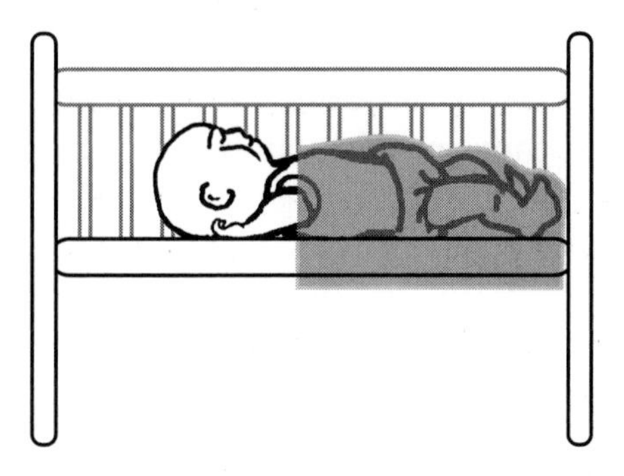

Figure 45 Feet to foot position

It is important not to restrict the baby's ability to lose heat when hot and therefore hats and extra clothing should be removed whenever the baby is brought inside. The room temperature should be comfortable, about 18°C.

Breast feeding

Breast feeding should be encouraged wherever possible. It has many benefits and few disadvantages.

OTHER FACTORS

It is recommended that babies do not sleep in bed with their parents. Parents, and others who are entrusted with the care of infants, should be encouraged to seek medical advice promptly if an infant is unwell or thought to be unwell.

Recommended guidance to parents and others who have responsibility for the care of infants (taken from the Report of the Chief Medical Officer's Expert Group on the Sleeping Position of Infants and Cot Deaths):

- The room where an infant sleeps should be at a temperature which is comfortable for lightly clothed adults, i.e. 16–20°C.
- When indoors, infants need little more bedding than adults.
- Bedding should not be excessive for the temperature of the room.
- Bedding should be arranged so that the infant is unlikely to slip underneath; for example, it can be made up so that the infant's feet come down to the end of the cot.
- Duvets should not be used for an infant under the age of one year.
- Bedding should not be increased when the infant is unwell or feverish.
- An infant should not be exposed to direct heating whilst asleep, for example from a hot-water bottle, electric blanket radiant heater.
- An infant over one month, at home, does not need to be kept as warm as in the hospital baby nursery.
- An infant over one month of age should not wear hats indoors for sleeping, unless the room is very cold.
- When infants are taken outdoors in cold weather they chill rapidly, and it is essential that they are adequately wrapped.

IF A COT DEATH OCCURS

The carer who has found the baby may start artificial resuscitation (see page 188). An ambulance and doctor should be called. The doctor will certify that a cot death has occurred.

SUPPORT FOR THE CARERS AFTER A COT DEATH HAS OCCURRED

The parents will be told that a post-mortem will be necessary and that if the cause of death cannot be explained, it will be registered as a sudden infant death (a post-mortem is carried out on any person who dies unexpectedly). The parents should be allowed to say goodbye to the child. They should be allowed to hold her and be given privacy during this time.

The coroner will arrange for an inquest, and the parents may be asked to identify the child. The police will require statements from the parents; this is the usual procedure for any unexpected death. Once the death is registered, the funeral arrangements will be made. The doctor and health visitor will help and support the family during this time. The mother may need advice on the suppression of lactation. The parents will probably want to talk and ask questions. They will require time from various professionals. The siblings must also be considered, as they too will grieve for the baby (see page 208).

Parents should be told about 'normal grief' and its pattern. There are several self-help groups that they may be put in touch with. The role of the early years worker must not be forgotten; although not necessarily a relative, she may be very close to the infant, especially if she is the nanny. The health visitor will call and often provide a sympathetic ear. Sometimes the parents may need extra help and support with other children.

ACTIVITY

You are working in a day nursery. Although you are not in charge, you take part in the induction of nursery nurse students for their work experience. You have been asked to prepare a teaching session lasting for twenty minutes on the safety of sleeping babies.

You will need to allow time to find out what the students already know about the subject. How will you go about finding out? (Perhaps you will ask questions and respond to answers? Perhaps you will prepare some written questions requiring short answers?)

You will need to cover the most important aspects of safety in this session, but will need to build on the information in subsequent sessions. What information do you think you will need to feed back to your supervisor?

Conclusion

Caring for a child with a terminal illness can be an exacting and yet fulfilling experience for the carer, knowing that she has done all she can to help and support the child and her parents at this time. However, it can also be a harrowing experience and the carer may find that she needs support. If this is the case she should perhaps approach her general practitioner who may suggest that she sees a counsellor.

Conclusion

Child carers are in a very privileged position: they have made a career out of looking after other people's children and it can be a most rewarding and fulfilling occupation. No two days are the same; children bring with them their infectious curiosity and enthusiasm for life. Few occupations carry greater responsibilities. The carer is a role model for children in her care and as such she has a responsibility to ensure that she sets a good example and provides the children with the right experiences to learn about and adopt a healthy lifestyle. She must be 'in tune' with her charges at all times and ready to notice the slight differences that might suggest illness. In order to do this, she needs to have the confidence and the knowledge to cope with the situation.

This book set out to provide the underpinning knowledge but learning should not stop here. The carer is a professional who must be aware of new developments in the field, including developments in child health. Individuals must accept the responsibility of keeping themselves up to date with changes; this can be done through courses run by colleges, or social services and also through discussions with others in the field, reading specialised magazines and books such as this one.

Glossary

allergy – occurs when a foreign substance enters the body and causes the immune system to over-react in a harmful way
aminoacid – the end-product of protein digestion
antibodies – a substance which the body produces in response to an antigen
antigen – a substance which stimulates the production of antibodies
aorta – the artery that leaves the left side of the heart
appendix – a blind-ended tube leading from the large intestine
ataxic – loss of power governing movements, usually refers to walking
auroscope – an instrument used by a doctor to examine the middle ear
bilirubin – the breakdown product of red blood cells
cardiac sphincter – muscular tissue where the oesophagus meets the stomach
cataract – an opacity of the lens of the eye which prevents light reaching the back of the eye
cerebro-spinal fluid – fluid bathing the brain and spinal cord, found also in the ventricles of the brain
congenital – born with
convulsion – uncontrolled movements of muscles which may be accompanied by a loss of consciousness
cytotoxic medication – a medication that damages cells and is used in the treatment of cancer
diagnosis – identification of the cause of disease by the patient's symptoms
diphtheria – a bacterial infection in the throat, in which a grey membrane may form over the tonsils causing a blockage. The bacteria produce toxins which may affect the heart and the nerves. Rarely seen in Britain these days because of the effective immunisation programme
ductus arteriosus – the blood vessel that connects the pulmonary artery and the aorta in the foetus; the blood therefore by-passes the lungs. It usually closes at or soon after birth
electro encephalogram (EEG) – an instrument used to measure the electrical currents produced in the brain
empower – to enable
enzyme – substance that accelerates the breakdown of food for absorption
exacerbation – worsening of the condition, demonstrated by signs and symptoms
febrile convulsion – uncontrolled movements of muscles; may be accompanied by loss of consciousness, associated with raised temperature
femoral pulse – a pulse felt in the groin where the femoral artery runs down the leg. The pulse at the top of each leg should be of similar strength
five-year survival rate – the percentage of people living five years after the diagnosis of a cancer
glue ear – fluid behind the ear drum causing partial deafness

histology – the study of the structures of tissues
HIV – human immunodeficiency virus
hydrocephalus – an excess of cerebro-spinal fluid around the brain resulting in a large head
immunisation – induction of immunity against bacterial or viral agents
incubation period – the time between being infected and the appearance of signs and symptoms
invasive – the destruction of healthy tissue by a malignant tumour
jaundice – yellow coloration of the skin and sclera (white of the eye) caused by the interference with the production of bile
ketones – the breakdown product of fat metabolism
low birth weight – a baby born weighing less than five pounds in weight
meninges – the protective coverings of the brain and spinal cord
neurosurgeon – a surgeon who specialises in surgery to the brain and nerves
nucleus – the central part of the cell
nystagmus – fine jerky movements of the eyes which are involuntary
ophthalmoscope – an instrument used to examine the back of the eye
premature – a baby born less than thirty-seven weeks after the first day of the last menstrual period
poliomyelitis (polio) – a viral infection affecting the nervous system. Rarely seen in Britain these days because of effective immunisation
prognosis – the probable result of a disease
pyloric sphincter – the muscular tissue that controls the passage of the stomach contents into the small intestine
remission – lessening of the effects of the disease and possibly the temporary disappearance of the signs and symptoms
retinoblastoma – a rare tumour of the retina
rib recession – where the muscles between the ribs are sucked in (may be seen in asthma)
salivary glands – these are situated near the mouth and secrete saliva. They include the parotid gland, the sublingual gland and the submaxillary gland
space blanket – a foil blanket designed to prevent further heat loss when used as per instructions
syndrome – a combination of signs and/or symptoms which suggest a specific disorder
tetanus (lockjaw) – a bacterial infection in which the muscles of the jaw and neck go into spasm. Rarely seen in Britain these days because of the effective immunisation programme
toddler – a child between the ages of one and two-and-a-half years of age
tonsillectomy – removal of the tonsils
trimester – a third of the time spent in pregnancy
vernix – the waxy substance that protects the skin of newborn babies
vesicles – small, fluid-filled blisters

Care and Education Courses – Linking Courses to Units

NNEB DIPLOMA MODULES	BTEC UNITS	NVQ CORE UNIT
M	1042L	C2
G		E2

Useful Addresses

Action for Sick Child
Argyle House
29–31 Euston Road
London
NW1 2SD
Helpline tel: 0171 833 2041
Admin tel: 0171 822 2041
Admin fax: 0171 837 2110

Anaphylaxis Campaign
PO Box 149
Fleet
Hampshire
GU13 9XU
Admin tel: 01252 318723

Association for Children with Heart Disorders, The
Killieard House
Killiecrankie
Pitlochry
Perthshire
PH16 5LN
Helpline tel: 01796 473204
Admin tel: 01796 473204

Association for Children with Life-Threatening or Terminal Conditions and their families (ACT)
65 St Michael's Hill
Bristol
BS2 8DZ
Admin tel: 0117 922 1556
Admin fax: 0117 930 4707

Association for Spina Bifida And Hydrocephalus (ASBAH)
ASBAH House
42 Park Road
Peterborough
PE1 2UQ
Admin tel: 01733 555988
Admin fax: 01733 555985

AVERT (AIDS Education and Research Trust, The)
11 Denne Parade
Horsham
West Sussex
RH12 1JD
Admin tel: 01403 210202
Admin fax: 01403 211001

British Diabetic Association
10 Queen Anne Street
London
W1M 0BD
Tel: 0171 323 1531

British Epilepsy Association
Anstey House
40 Hanover Square
Leeds
LS3 1BE
Helpline tel: 0800 309030
Admin tel: 0113 243 9393
Admin fax: 0113 242 8804

Cancer and Leukaemia In Childhood (CLIC)
12–13 King Square
Bristol
BS2 8JH
Helpline tel: 0117 924 8844
Admin tel: 0117 924 8844
Admin fax: 0117 924 4505

Child Accident Prevention Trust
4th Floor
18–20 Farringdon Lane
London
EC1R 3AU
Admin tel: 0171 608 3828
Admin fax: 0171 608 3674

Child Growth Foundation
2 Mayfield Avenue
Chiswick
London
W4 1PW
Helpline tel: 0181 995 0257
Admin tel: 0181 995 0257
Admin fax: 0181 995 9075

Cleft Lip And Palate Association (CLAPA)
134 Buckingham Palace Road
London
SW1 9SA
Admin tel: 0171 824 8110
Admin fax: 0171 824 8109

Coeliac Society, The
PO Box 220
High Wycombe
Bucks
HP11 2HY
Helpline tel: 01494 437278
Admin fax: 01494 474349

Cruse – Bereavement Centre
126 Sheen Road
Richmond
Surrey
TW9 1UR
Tel: 0181 940 4818

Down's Syndrome Association
155 Mitcham Road
London
SW17 9PG
Helpline tel: 0181 682 4001
Admin tel: 0181 682 4001
Admin fax: 0181 682 4012

Foundation for the Study of Infant Deaths, The
14 Halkin Street
London
SW1X 7DP
Helpline tel: 0171 235 1721
Admin tel: 0171 235 0965
Admin fax: 0171 823 1986

Health Education Authority
Hamilton House
Mabledon Place
London
WC1H 9JP
Admin tel: 0171 383 3833

Meningitis Research Foundation
13 High Street
Thornbury
Bristol
BS12 2AE
Helpline tel: 01454 413344
Admin tel: 01454 281811
Admin fax: 01454 281094

National Asthma Campaign
Providence House
Providence Place
London
N1 0NT
Helpline tel: 0345 010203
Admin tel: 0171 226 2260
Admin fax: 0171 704 1740

National Ezcema Society
163 Eversholt Street
London
NW1 1BU
Helpline tel: 0171 388 4800
Admin tel: 0171 388 5651
Admin fax: 0171 388 5882

National Meningitis Trust
Fern House
Bath Road
Stroud
Gloucestershire
GL5 3TJ
Helpline tel: 0345 538118
Admin tel: 01453 751738
Admin fax: 01453 753588

National Society for Epilepsy, The
Information Department
Chalfont St Peter
Gerrards Cross
Buckinghamshire
SL9 0RJ
Helpline tel: 01494 601400/873991
Admin tel: 01494 601300/873991
Admin fax: 01494 871927

NSPCC
42 Curtain Road
London
EC2A 3NH
Helpline tel: 0800 800500
Admin tel: 0171 825 2775
Admin fax: 0171 825 2763

Scope
12 Park Crescent
London
W1N 4EQ
Helpline tel: 0800 626216
Admin tel: 0171 636 5020
Admin fax: 0171 436 2601

Sickle Cell Society
54 Station Road
Harlesden
London
NW10 4UA
Admin tel: 0181 961 7995/961 4006
Admin fax: 0181 961 8346

Bibliography and References

Baggot, B. (1994) *Health and Health Care in Britain.* Macmillan, London.
Barnes, A. (1987) *Personal and Community Health.* Bailliere Tindall, London.
Bee, H. (1992) *The Developing Child.* HarperCollins, London.
BMA (1990) *The Complete Family Encyclopaedia.* Dorling Kindersley, London.
Bowlby, J. (1975) *Attachment and Loss Vol. 1 Attachment.* Pelican, Harmondsworth.
Bruce, T. and Meggitt, C. (1996) *Child Care and Education.* Hodder and Stoughton, London.
Coffey, J. (1995) *Care of the Sick Child.* Hodder and Stoughton, London.
DfEE (1996) *Supporting Pupils with Medical Needs.* Crown Copyright, UK.
DHSS (1976) *Prevention and Health – everybody's business.* HMSO, London.
DHSS (1980) *Inequalities in Health. Report of a research working group to the DHSS (The Black Report).* HMSO, London.
DHSS (1988) *Present Day Practice in Infant Feeding: Third Report.* HMSO, London.
DOH (1989) *The Children Act.* HMSO, London.
DOH (1991) *Welfare of Children and Young People in Hospital.* HMSO, London.
DOH (1993) *The Sleeping Position of Infants and Cot Death.* HMSO, London.
DOH (1992) *The Health of the Nation.* HMSO, London.
DOH (1996) *Immunisation against Infectious Disease.* HMSO, London.
Ewles, L. and Simnett, I. (1992) *Promoting Health: A Practical Guide to Health Education.* Scutari Press, London.
Felscher, H. (ed.) (1993) *Stedman's Pocket Dictionary.* Williams and Wilkins, London.
Furley, A. (1989) *A Bad Start in Life – Children, Health and Housing.* Shelter Publications.
Hall, D.M.B. (ed.) (1996) *Health for All Children.* Oxford University Press, Oxford.
Hilton, T. (1991) *The Great Ormond Street Book of Baby and Child Care.* The Bodley Head, London.
Jones, H. (1996) *Your Child's Health.* Hodder and Stoughton, London.
Kempe, R. and Kempe, H. (1978) *Child Abuse.* Fontana, London.
Landsdown, R. (1996) *Children in Hospital.* Oxford University Press, Oxford.
Levene, S. (1992) *Play it Safe.* BBC Books, London.
Lewer, H. and Robertson, L. (1983) *Care of the Child.* Macmillan, London.

Lwin, R., Duggan, C. and Gibb, D. (1993) *HIV and AIDS in Children: A Guide for the Family.* The Hospitals for Sick Children, The Institute of Child Health.

Morton, J. and Macfarlane, A. (1991) *Child Health and Surveillance.* Blackwell Scientific Publications, Oxford.

Minett, P., Wayne, D. and Rubenstein, D. (1989) *Human Form and Function.* Unwin Hyman, London.

Naidoo, J. and Wills, J. (1994) *Health Promotion.* Bailliere Tindall, London.

O'Hagan, M. and Smith, M. (1993) *Special Issues in Child Care.* Bailliere Tindall, London.

Parker, M. and Stucke, V. (1987) *Microbiology for Nurses.* Bailliere Tindall, London.

Robertson, J. and J. (1976) *Young Children in Brief Separation: a guide to the film series.* The Robertson Centre, London.

Rodin, J. (1983) *Will This Hurt?* R.C.N., London.

Sheridan, M. (1992) *From Birth to Five.* Routledge, London.

St John's Ambulance (1992) *First Aid Manual.* Dorling Kindersley, London.

Stoppard, M. (1991) *Baby and Child Health Handbook.* Dorling Kindersley, London.

Townsend, P. and Davidson, N. (eds.) in Whitehead, M. (1988) *Inequalities in Health: The Black Report and The Health Divide.* Penguin, London.

Weller, B. (1980) *Helping Sick Children Play.* Bailliere Tindall, London.

Whalley Wong (1983) *Nursing Care of Infants and Young Children.* Mosby St Louis, USA.

Wolfe, L. (1993) *Safe and Sound.* Hodder and Stoughton, London.

Youngston, R.M. (1995) *The Royal Society of Medicine Encyclopaedia of Family Health.* Bloomsbury, London.

Index